Comments from early readers:

"I wish I had read this in my younger life!…This is so informational <u>and</u> entertaining to read – I feel like I have a guide through life's difficulties when I read this."

(Erika D)

Deborah,

Thank you. Thanks again for sharing this. I have needed this message for so long. You are such a blessing to me and others. I am so touched by your wisdom and insight…Your work on mental illness helps me every day. I have been reading it again; it is helping me.

(Monica B)

I thought it very useful to those who have psychiatric problems, and I felt your writing was great. I just wanted to keep reading and find out what came next and what could be done to deal with the problems involved.

(Donna W)

Something that is so valuable, a compilation of personal experience, personal advice, and Twelve-Step guidance that offers real, effective ideas for dealing with the crap that goes with mental illness. I wish I had time now to elaborate and tell you all the things I liked, but that will have to wait. For now just know I LOVE this, I'm looking forward to having a copy of it, and these last three chapters I'm going to sit and read with my husband.

(Kathy D)

Room For Me, Too, made me see that there is, indeed, room for me and for all of us. It showed me that we all matter, and that we've been lost because we never had a place to start. Deborah offers her readers a place to begin and holds their hand along the way. She picks you up and seems to say, "There you go, try this...I did it and you can too."

Room For Me, Too, is bravely honest and heartfelt. I have read a lot of non-fiction and this is the first time I would call a book a true work of humanity. Her interviews are the most complete and caring I have ever seen before. Even the religious parts were a huge breath of fresh air...None of us are without issues, and I can't think of anyone who wouldn't benefit greatly from this book. This book was intended for those with mental illnesses of various types, but I say it's a must read for those who know anyone with such problems.

(Leslie D)

IS THERE ROOM FOR ME, TOO?

-- Twelve Steps & Twelve Strategies for Coping with Mental Illness

Written by Deborah Fruchey

with an introduction by Dr. David Kallinger
section on world religions by Mel C. Thompson
photography by Robert Hamaker

With abundant thanks to my amazing husband,
whose support, encouragement, and technical savvy made this
book immensely richer

ISBN 1450596843
ISBN-13 9781450596848
Library of Congress Control Number: 2010907392

DEDICATED

TO ROSE,
WHO FIGURED IT OUT

TO RUBEN,
WHO MADE IT BETTER

TO NANCY,
WHO MADE IT WORK

AND
TO ALL THOSE BELOVED SOULS
WHO DIDN'T MAKE IT

CONTENTS

Foreword

Suppose you go to work one day, and the walls start talking to you.

You'd like to ignore them. But they are saying things you've secretly suspected for years.

You go to a doctor. He sends you to a psychiatrist. The psychiatrist gives you pills, which he tells you may or may not take care of it. Make another appointment. Plan to do this for life, because the prognosis is not good. Then he sends you home.

What now?

What do you tell your family? What do you tell your employer (if you still even have an employer)? What do you tell your friends?

What do you tell yourself?

This happens to millions of people a year. But I have yet to see a book that tells you what to do next. Nobody told me.

What this book has to offer you is 36 years of experience on what to do next.

My personal plan of action comes from the Twelve Steps made famous by Alcoholics Anonymous. This is not because I equate mental illness with addiction – I don't. It's in part because I spent a lot of years in that association. I am no longer attending those meetings or living exactly by those rules. But I find them a very potent method for kick-starting a life that isn't working.

The language is old-fashioned, but the principles are psychologically sound. There are probably lots of other ways to structure a fulfilling life as a psychiatric patient. My experience shows that this method works. The Twelve Steps are a great way to re-boot a life that has somehow gone drastically off in the wrong direction.

But this is not just another Twelve Step book. Each chapter has a Twelve-Step, 'Inner Person' section, yes ~ and a practical, 'Outer Person' section containing the tips and tricks I've learned over the decades. I call these the Twelve Strategies, though there are far more than twelve seeded throughout the text. You will find out how to navigate your way through bureaucracies and services; who to tell and what to tell them; ways to deal with psychosis; how to survive suicidal thoughts; and more.

You can skip straight to the practical section if you wish (but don't miss the hard-core advice in Step 10). The Strategies encompass virtually everything I have learned in over 30 years of living with abnormal psychology, and a good deal more that my interview subjects suggested.

Of course any book has limitations. There are certain things you won't find here, and it's only fair to note them.

For instance: this is not program-approved material. It has not been through any formal approval process by any Twelve-Step councils or members. Some people won't like that.

But I can't find anyone out there talking to the mentally ill about handling life's daily issues. It needs to be done.

Another point I must make: I am not a psychological expert. I am only an educated layman who has subjected her book to rigorous oversight by the kind and generous Dr. David Kallinger. His education and clinical expertise will hopefully cover any gaps where my experience might fail. And I know that there are places where I must necessarily fall short. For instance, I am Bipolar with Psychotic Features. If you have some other disorder, such as Schizophrenia, or Panic Disorder, you may not find quite as much material or detail as you would like. I have consulted as many people with as many different conditions as I was able, though.

Reading this book is not a substitute for proper medical care. Nothing in this book should be construed as medical advice.

On the other hand, don't you think we've heard enough from the 'experts'? What do they really know about living with a brain that *lies* to you? What do they know about living on Disability, or shame, or the fear you'll never work again? Have you read some of those authoritative manuals? They make mental illness sound minor and quaint, like missing one finger from a non-dominant hand. Those of us who've been there know better. We need a lot more than pictures of abnormal brain cells, and triple-jointed medical terms.

In this spectrum of diseases I'd like to include, by mention, the victims of other 'invisible illnesses'. These people are exposed to similar bias and ignorance. The emotional and life stresses can be very similar. Such invisible diseases include

Chronic Fatigue Syndrome (whatever medical label it eventually falls under), Multiple Sclerosis in its earlier stages, certain degrees of legal blindness, Lupus, and any number of other problems. They can restrict and reshape a life but aren't visible to the eyes. I want to offer my recognition and support to these additional brothers and sisters.

There is NO substitute for consistent, diligent, individually appropriate care. It is up to you to find the right doctor, the right therapist, the right health routines, the right safeguards. *Whatever it takes.* To live decently with a neurobiological illness takes as much dedication and courage as fighting drug addiction. It is a full-time job. You must participate.

I repeat. Don't skimp on the medicine and expect the program to bail you out.

I feel so strongly about this! It's so important!

In fact, if you're not willing to take proper medical care, I recommend you close this book and go home right now. I mean it. Go home and have a few more disasters, and then come back when you're ready to do the work.

A word about alternate and holistic care: I think mind/body medicine is wonderful. If you are in the forefront and willing to give these things a chance, more power to you. I would not discourage anyone from availing themselves of vitamin therapy, or traditional Chinese medicine, or shiatsu, or sound therapy, or Bach flower essences. But be aware that these things are not covered by most insurance, including Medicare and Medicaid, so they are going to be expensive. The government will not accept them as 'medical treatment' in most cases, so you will be ineligible for benefits. Thirdly, my experience is that these remedies are mild, and slow to make a difference. When we are first dealing with powerful symptoms that make chaos of our lives, we need immediate, powerful relief. When it comes to fast, measurable results, there is still nothing like Western (allopathic) medicine. I would suggest a combination that moves gradually from one to the other in a slow arc.

But if you're willing to work on your health, then it's time to look at the Steps and Strategies I explain here. Mental illness may be the end of life as you've known it, *but it is not the end of your life.* There is so much more available than mere survival!

I have a favorite quote, from the <u>Sex and Love Addicts Anonymous</u> handbook (yes, I've been in that program, too). It says, "The truth is, we feel we are on to something big. We don't know where it will lead us. *We just don't know what the upper limits of healthy human functioning are*" (italics mine).

I know there are lots of you out there. I know we need each other. Reach with me, up into the dark.

Deborah Fruchey

SOME BASIC INFORMATION
        By Dr. David M. Kallinger

PROLOGUE:

This is a description of psychiatric diagnostic categories. Let me begin by stating that every psychiatric diagnosis exists within every person. Everyone is depressed, anxious, ruminates, and has unusual thoughts. The major difference between "normal" people and those with mental illness has to do with degree. People who are mentally ill are more depressed, more anxious, ruminate more, and have more unusual thinking. These symptoms tend to interfere with their lives and make it harder to concentrate and go to school, have careers, succeed in relationships, etc.

Because most everyone does have some sort of psychiatric symptom, and actually most everyone has all of the different symptoms mentioned above, it is sometimes hard to actually come up with a diagnosis. In my early days working with people that have mental illness, a wise psychiatrist who was a consultant to an agency where I worked said that it is best to diagnose someone early in the process of working with them. Otherwise, this man emphasized that the longer you would see someone, the more you would see the numerous psychiatric diagnoses in everyone. His point is actually true even for those of us who are being trained as psychologists, for we start believing that we have every psychiatric diagnosis that we study. As you familiarize yourself with a particular diagnosis, often you take on that diagnosis or at least see aspects of it in your own personality. It can be exhausting to study the various mental health conditions for one feels that one becomes all of them.

Now that we have some of the introductory statements out of the way, let me outline for you what will follow. I will articulate a model that will categorize the various diagnoses into major components. This model will suggest that mental illness falls into identified groups. These consist of Anxiety related Disorders, Disorders of thought processes, and finally those of mood. There are Personality Disorders which, for the most part, fall into the previously mentioned schema so will not be separately described.

So now that I have laid out these categories, is my job done? (Well, gee, I am feeling too anxious to continue, my thoughts are foggy, and my mood is in the dumps...I can't go on any further! I need to rest my case!)

If only it were so simple! But alas, it is not, so I will continue.

ANXIETY REACTIONS:

Anxiety is the first category which we will review. Anxiety is experienced both psychically as fear or a pervasive sense of unwellness, and felt physically in the body (e.g., the digestive tract). Anxiety can be either "free floating" or directly connected to certain events. When it is free floating, it can be experienced as trepidation or an impending sense of disaster: a predilection that an ominous event is about to occur. Anxiety can be triggered by specific sequences of stimuli such as crowds, heights, dirt, animal hair, etc. When it is attached to various stimuli, fear often results. We may not know that what we are afraid of will happen, but we are convinced that something will harm us. Therefore, 'attachment to a stimuli' means a defensive attempt at prevention. That is, we avoid crowds, or heights, or the sun, or whatever we fear. The idea is to engage in certain routines, known as rituals, to help stave off the feared result that we expect. Most of the time we do not know what is really being avoided.

Anxiety related conditions include Generalized Anxiety, Phobias, and Obsessive-Compulsive Disorders; people who "cut" themselves or pull out their hair (Trichotillomania). The Anxiety response, defensive in nature, is very often either physiological -- related to the body -- or triggered by outside events such as crowds, heights. People with Obsessive-Compulsive conditions engage in rituals to stave off the feared result: touching door knobs before leaving a room or house, always driving the same routes without fail, engaging in ritualized behaviors before stepping into the batting box as a batter in a baseball game. To some extent we all engage in rituals but not to the extent that they rule our lives. Most people do not hold objects over their heads to avoid the sun striking their skin. In that instance, the ritualized behavior is to avoid getting older. This brings me around to stating that I believe that most all anxieties are at their root connected to the fear of death.

THOUGHT DISORDERS:

Now let us look at the second category of diagnosing people with mental impairments. This area has to do with thought processes. That is, simply put, how do we think? Thinking is aligned with reality, what is actually occurring in the world. Now, granted, perceptions are a factor in reality. People can perceive reality from their own perspective. I have heard it said that you can get five different opinions from five people who witness an automobile accident, depending on their frame of reference or past experience. Generally speaking, we can derive certain facts that occur that most people will agree happened and we call this reality. In the realm of the psychological, this can become more difficult.

As a general rule, there are perceptions which are seen as abnormal, that is, out of the range that most people experience. Here we are talking about hallucinations and delusions. Some people see and hear persons and events that the majority of us would say do not exist.

This can be complicated even further when it comes to religious doctrines and experiences. I am told that people have "visions" of certain religious figures. Most of the time these are single occurrences. No doubt those religious beliefs have tremendous appeal to certain individuals, prescribing doctrines which attempt to regulate human behavior. One result of such strong prescriptions is to identify right and wrong ways of acting. This tends to lead people into feeling guilty when they do not live up to such doctrines. Some of these beliefs have to do with sexual behavior, which is a very strong trigger for guilt and shame. I remember visiting a friend of mine in the 1960's who was finishing his studies to be a Baptist pastor and was assigned, as part of his training, to work in a state mental hospital. I recall that most of the inhabitants displayed unusual behaviors, e.g., standing against walls with their arms outstretched as if they were Jesus on the cross, or many women wearing white clothes claiming to be Mary, the virgin mother.

It is necessary to talk about the opposition of fantasy and reality. Fantasy exists within our minds. We can have prescriptions for life which originate, or at least are exemplified, by fantasies. I may believe, for instance, that I have some very sordid sexual proclivities, because my father told me that I was a whore in my teenage years. My perceptions of what my father told me could have been affected by my own raging hormones, and I certainly wouldn't understand my father's fears at such a young age. Therefore, I may have this fantasy, fueled to some extent by events in the world in my youth, that I am a horrible sexual deviant. Because of these beliefs I could punish myself by acting in sexually seductive ways and believing that people's reactions to me are at their root due to my dirty, sexual thoughts. There actually may not be any reality to my dilemma and the partial truths may not really have any bases in the world.

The diagnostic category of Thought Disorders are exhibited in such conditions as Schizophrenia or Paranoid thinking. To reach the diagnostic criteria necessary for Schizophrenia, someone must have very obvious lapses in reality which can be exemplified by hallucinations (visions or hearing voices) or by delusions, beliefs that really have no bases in reality (e.g., I will remain youthful if I enter into a trance at age 17).

Sometimes breaks with reality are temporary or short term, while other beliefs are quite fixed. I can believe that my sexual proclivities result in a group of people constantly assailing me and exposing my sexuality. In Paranoid thinking, the person takes feelings that they have about themselves and projects these out on to other people.

The classic example in psychological annals is in reaction formation, when very straight-laced women stand outside of sex shows with signs decrying the exhibition of such explicit sexual activities, while these same very proper women have their own hidden sexual fantasies and exhibitionistic tendencies. It is not safe to feel the emotions directly so we externalize these feelings on to other people and blame them. I know of a very angry man who projects out his own self-hatred on to political figures and family members whom he sees as being very harsh and lacking in understanding. To some extent, these externalized figures represent his critical father.

In summary, once again, we all have odd or unusual thought patterns, but when these get in our way and prevent us from interacting and functioning in the world, then they become distinct liabilities. Also in the realm of Obsessive-Compulsive Disorders, you probably have picked up that symptoms of Anxiety and Thought Disorder come together to form ritualized behavior. We will also observe this blending of categories in our next and final description.

MOOD DISORDERS:

Most of us are familiar with slightly depressed moods as well as increased productive cycles accompanied by elevated moods which would be classified as Manic in nature. People with mental illness experience these two polar opposite affects -- Depression and Mania -- in rather large doses. As is the way of human experience, it is very difficult to come up with a profile that fits everyone. Some people have very prolonged Depressions with suicidal thoughts, a sense of hopelessness, a pessimistic outlook on the world, loss of appetite and disturbed sleep cycles. Depressions can go on for long periods of time in relentless fashion with very little reprieve. Others have very deep downward mood periods which last for short spans of time. Then there are people who have less profound down cycles which impair functioning in the world but the symptoms are more measured. Of course, individuals can display anything between these two extremes. Hence the term Dysthymia, which corresponds with minor Depressive symptoms, and Major Depression, which can have periods of loss of contact with reality. People tend to experience Depression both on a physiological level, and on the physical - the sense of being weighed down in one's body, lack of appetite, lowered sex drive, interference with sleep patterns, etc. Depression is also experienced psychically as hopelessness, despair, pessimism, low self-esteem, and a feeling that one will fail at whatever one sets out to accomplish. So we observe a blending of the psychological and physiological in downward mood swings.

Medication can help with Depressive symptoms but most of the time does not eradicate the lowered mood. We know that exercise helps. Most of the time Depressed people blame themselves for their deflated mood but some people believe their Depression is caused by others or outside circumstances.

On the opposite end of affective responses is Mania. As with Depression, there are deviations between slight mood elevation and soaring grandiosity. I once knew a single, poor woman who had two children and in a Manic phase convinced a car dealer to lease her a very expensive automobile; then she got work at an Ethan Allen store selling high-end furniture. When she came down from the Manic state, it was impossible to keep the high-stress job and pay for her car, so this woman returned to welfare payments to survive.

In a Manic period, one can feel capable of taking on the world, can have very grandiose assessments of their abilities, and can actually perform at very high levels. Often such phases are accompanied by lack of need for sleep, agitation, and irritability. There are very successful literary and artistic historical figures who are believed to have been Manic-Depressive. We know that the difference between sanity and insanity can be a slight degree. There seems to be little doubt that major accomplishments have occurred while certain people have been Manic. In such instances the mind appears to harness tremendous energy to create outstanding results. Mania can be one vehicle to reach such psychic levels.

Most people are aware of a Bipolar diagnosis. This is the old Manic-Depressive syndrome which got far more attention after the development of lithium. As is the case with most diagnostic categories, Bipolar conditions vary widely. Some people exhibit more Unipolar episodes, mainly Depression. Other people have numerous Manic phases and exhibit few Depressive episodes. Others have rapid cycling between Depression and Mania, sometimes up to six cycles in one day.

For the most part, current research suggests that Bipolar conditions are biochemical and possibly genetic, that they are passed on from one family member to another. Medication is the predominant approach to treatment. There is no single Bipolar medication. Usually psychiatrists put together different regimes of medications based on individual profiles.

A prominent diagnosis these days is Schizo-Affective Disorder. This is a combination of a Thought Disorder along with a mood condition. So, once again, we observe a blending effect between the different categories. Mood Disorders receive much attention these days and we are discovering more about how they exhibit and what treatment modalities work to minimize symptoms. Affects, or emotions, are central to our human experience. We attempt to alter our mood by the use of alcohol or drugs. People with Bipolar diagnosis have no choice in the matter and the goal is more to help these people modulate their emotions.

SUMMARY:

We have reached the end of our road in describing the basic categories of mental illness. I remind you that mental disease symptoms exist in all of us in a modulated form. People with mental health issues who display Anxiety, thought distortions, and mood swings typically do so in exaggerated ways which interfere with their ability to function in the world. We all have fantasies that compete with our sense of reality. When these internal scenarios take over our lives and predominate, then we lose contact with reality. Many of these fantasies at their roots have to do with fears of dying, our own sexuality, feelings of self-worth, and attachments to those around us. We tend to blame ourselves for events that go wrong and feel guilty over events when we take too much credit for their actual outcomes.

We know more these days about mental illness, and connections are being made daily combining mental functioning with the brain. There has been some improvement in how we treat mental illness. We no longer put people away in institutions and ignore them. We understand mental aberrations better and accept those of us who suffer from them. There still is a belief that mental illness is self-induced, that those who have it are complicit in some way for their condition. We believe that people with emotional issues are unstable and can act out against society. The evidence is that most people with mental illness act out against themselves, not others. We know that physiological manifestations have real impact on emotional functioning. In fact we now know that there is a constant interchange occurring between the mind and the body.

Developmentally, we understand that infantile reactions are at the root of emotional functioning. We know that the ability to symbolize - that is, to exhibit physiological responses and transfer them into mental emotions - is a tremendous step in development. There is a constant interchange between the mental and the bodily. Continued research is showing more convincingly that physiological decline can directly result from mental symptoms. People who are lonely and depressed tend to deteriorate faster physically. We try to harness our loneliness and lack of sense of community by the use of alcohol and both illegal and legal drugs, including antidepressants.

This, according to Dean Ornish, is an attempt to avoid the universal pain inherent in life. We do not have the strong ties to family and community as in the past, so we disappear into large cities and suffer alone. Alas, if we cannot have empathy for our own plight then how can we understand those among us who display mental illness? They remind us of what we feel are our own failings. There is a need for more understanding and empathy if we hope to calm the raging impulses that exist within the human psyche.

PART ONE:

THE SEARCH FOR SANITY

I don't fear none of my enemies
And I don't fear bullets from uzis
I been dealing with something that's
Worse than these
That makes you fall to your knees
And that's my anxieties.
- "Anxiety" from Elephunk by the Black Eyed Peas

Who we are, what we want

People only hear about us when we kill somebody.

Remember Andrea Yates? She drowned all six of her kids in the bathtub during a desperate Depression. Or what about that woman who threw her three babies in San Francisco Bay, because a voice told her to? She still thinks she did a good thing. One of the scariest in the pantheon is Seung Hai Cho, who shot down 32 people at Virginia Tech. He didn't get enough treatment. It happens. And it gets in the news.

This is the image the public has of mental illness. Most people envision us in hospitals, running down the halls screaming; or in strait-jackets, wild-eyed, biting our attendants. Walking down city streets in ragged clothes mumbling to ourselves. Or sitting motionless in corners, old and hopeless, staring at walls and things which nobody else can see; speaking cryptically to imaginary people, and requiring constant supervision.

Television hasn't helped our public relations much. Hasn't everyone at some time watched, say, a sweaty, creepy guy with a knife, hanging around a subterranean parking garage? This kind of plot is the darling of the Late Night Saturday Movie. I suppose a crazy guy comes in handy when the writers run out of ideas.

The picture even gets reinforced in great literature: <u>Jane Eyre</u>, for example. Who could forget the first Mrs. Rochester? Upon losing her marbles for reasons unspecified, she gets shut up in the attic and turns into something resembling an orangutan. Except when she gets out to bite people and set their beds on fire. I read <u>Jane Eyre</u> over and over as a child. I loved it. I still do. But I'd also like to kick Charlotte Bronte around the block for what she did to the collective social image of the insane.

There *are* people like that, of course, which is one reason the stereotypes persist. It's a wide, wild world, and there's room out there on the fringes for almost anything.

Here's what most people don't know: the average percentage of violence among the mentally ill is lower than the average percentage of violence among the total population.[1] Dangerous criminals among the abnormal are the exception rather than the rule (Corrigan & Watson, 2005). Most of us turn our violence against ourselves, not against others.

It doesn't fit our paradigms. If a person does something that awful, they MUST be crazy, right? Crazy is the only explanation, isn't it? The frightening truth is that most violent crime is committed by individuals who have no mental illness. They are reasoning, 'sane' individuals who think this course of action makes *sense.*

That statistic wouldn't sell any papers, though. So you won't hear about it. As a psychology professor of mine liked to say, "Mental Patient Lives Quietly, Dies Peacefully" just doesn't work as a headline.

I'm not talking about the extreme cases, splashy as they are. For one thing, they are very small in number. They are beyond the scope of this book, though I'd like to point out that they are still people, not just 'cases.' Deeply afflicted people, whose suffering is beyond our ability to understand, certainly deserve better than to be classed with demons and goblins.

My subject is the functionally insane. You probably know quite a few of them.

Unless they've told you their story, you probably don't recognize them as such. They comprise <u>one in five</u> of the American population, at some time in their lives (according to the National Institute of Mental Health). They are Schizophrenic, Panic-Disordered, Bipolar. They are doctors. Lawyers. Grocery clerks. Homemakers, stockbrokers, students and salespeople. They are Dysthymic, Clinically Depressed,

---

[1] I read this little statistical gem in the standard study guides that Dr Kallinger used for his oral exams. This is not obscure information: it is available to every clinician getting ready to obtain his license.

Personality Disordered. They go to church[2], drive cars, raise children, pay taxes, fall in love.

They come from every race, religion, gender, age, and background. They occur in the best of families. They occur in the worst of families. They have occurred throughout all history, for no reason we know. And they all have one thing in common.

They would give almost anything to be well.

What We Can Actually Have

Medically, not a whole lot.

As far as science and medicine go at this time, there are theories , but precious few answers.

There are treatments and pills, there are therapies and protective laws (not many) and support groups. Some of them are wonderful. Some of them are so-so. Properly prescribed and applied in the right combination, they can make the difference between life in an institution or a relatively productive and satisfying life outside.

But they do not make anyone well.

This is something that the healthy have a habit of misunderstanding. They have the most irritating way, if you mention any difficulties, of tilting their heads to one side and saying, "But, gee, aren't there pills for that kind of thing nowadays?" If you are one of these, and are reading in an effort to understand someone you know, please pay the next statement close attention.

Ultimately, medicine[3] offers only relief of symptoms.

That's it. That's all. And sometimes it is an extremely

---

[2] This phrase is used generically here and meant to include synagogues, mosques, temples, and houses of worship of all faiths.

[3] Not only Western medicine. I was once told by an Ayurvedic practitioner that mental disease was caused by the stars at birth. Thus, it is inevitable and presumably incurable.

limited relief. Medicine cannot offer a cure, mostly because it doesn't know what's wrong in the first place.

Basic Assumptions

I'm working from several assumptions in this book, and we might as well nail them down now. There are also some working definitions that need to be set, just so we understand each other.

The first assumption is that most forms of mental illness are currently incurable. Some of us do have temporary conditions which eventually, with or without treatment, go away. Or we may have a condition for life. Either way, medicine does not 'cure' it – it helps us live through the symptoms.

But we don't 'get well' in the normal sense. We don't wake up one day and say, 'Thank god, that's over!' as if we'd had some simple growth surgically removed. It's more like we've gone into remission from cancer. We will always be at risk for recurrence. And we will always have a different outlook, once we've been on the dark side.

I am not talking about people who are going through a difficult time and are understandably depressed or upset. I'm talking about a medical condition.

My second assumption is about the causes of mental disorders. Please note I am speaking of *biological* causes, not spiritual ones, which are up to you to define.

Like many other diseases which used to be lumped in with 'madness' - epilepsy and diabetes are examples which spring to mind - it appears that these problems are transmitted genetically, at least in part.

Just as most career alcoholics tend to have family lines littered with 'drunks,' you will find the genealogy of many mental patients pocked, like a minefield, with Depressed grandfathers, mysterious suicides, or a famous Aunt Tillie who-ran-amok-and-had-to-be-put-away-don't-talk-about-her.

Pablo C., retired warehouse worker, poet, and photographer, is a good example. He was wrongly diagnosed as a Schizophrenic in his twenties and nearly died of treatment.

We'll be getting to that story in due course. But years later, due to personal research, he finally realized that he had Obsessive-Compulsive Disorder – witness the 170 boxes of collected flea market knick-knacks that had to be packed last time he moved! When he had put the pieces of his research together, he suddenly remembered an old aunt he had been curious about as a child.

> "There was, by gosh, on the other side of the family tree...my father's sister, my Aunt Maxine, [a] terrible Obsessive...she didn't like anyone visiting her home. But when anyone visited, each time after someone used the bathroom, she would clean it...I went over there once, and sitting on the stove was a great big huge canning pot...and I looked in there, I remember, the water was boiling. I thought, 'What in the world is going on?' When we got home, I asked my dad, I said, 'It looked like Aunt Maxine was boiling sheets!' He sort of said, 'Yeah, she does that to decontaminate them.'"

Then there is Lisa, a mischievous blonde mom from Alabama, who answered my enquiries this way:

> "I'm 'supposedly' Bi-polar...I've suffered from Anxiety for a long time. My daughter [has] a tentative diagnosis of Bipolar...and minor self-mutilation, which breaks my heart. I was raised by a Paranoid Schizophrenic...my brother has attempted suicide twice. The second time was in my house...so yeah, I definitely have a history."

Though the genetic patterns haven't been cracked yet, the evidence is pretty substantive. As in alcoholism, certain neurotransmitters are being over-or under-produced, improperly distributed, or otherwise failing to follow a normal path; the trick is to find medicines which in some way redirect this pattern. There are also physical structures in the brain that are different in people who are mentally ill from those who are not. It is not clear whether these cause the disease, or the disease causes them. They could even be caused by the medicines. (There is a great deal of research in this field; it is well beyond my abilities to summarize all of it.)

There is also the eternal question of 'Nature versus Nurture' to be considered (what I call the "all Mommy's fault theory"). This is a little more dicey. I do not have a hard and fast assumption on this topic. Certainly, we are all deeply and often permanently affected by what happens in our families and growing-up environments. And since special chemistry runs in families, where do you draw the line? If Papa was crazy, wouldn't being raised by him be enough to make you crazy, too?

We've been fed a lot of lines. Lisa told me about her childhood myths in the form of a third-person story:

> "The little girl's Daddy explained to her, one day when he seemed to be sober, that her Mama was ill because of some trauma that happened when she was little. He said the doctors had assured him that it was not hereditary. The little girl said, 'So that means we can't catch it?' Her father only nodded, with a slight smile."

I am taking a median position: that special chemistry is (often) a hereditary problem which (probably) involves some environmental triggers.

Bear in mind that even in those illnesses that are not said to have a physical component, we really just don't know. Yet. It is only very recently that any serious scientific attention has been paid to this field. While we're waiting for medicine to find the answers, it behooves all of us to treat each other with respect and compassion, no matter how odd some problems may look to us.

My colleague, Dr David Kallinger, thinks that my position is somewhat unbalanced: that nurture and environment are at least 50% of the answer. He writes that many of the 'new' conclusions concerning behavior had actually already been stated in the earlier psychoanalytic literature. And it is true that there are a number of other models to explain 'abnormal' psychology – cognitive, client-centered, gestalt, and psychodynamic, (which is David's specialty). I do not discard these at all. They are all helpful in terms of straightening out one's head. But they have only limited success in changing a lifetime illness. It is not the people with an event-triggered 'nervous breakdown' which goes away in six weeks or six months whom I am chiefly addressing, though I can hope to be helpful to them as well. I am talking about the people who receive the best Western medicine has to offer, and are still inarguably sick. I am talking about people for whom this is a way of life, at least for a year or two.

As for Nature and Nurture, David may well be correct. There is certainly evidence on both sides of this issue. Given that my father was Bipolar AND the head of the household, I cannot reasonably separate genetics from nurture in my own case. But the fact remains, under either theory, that the infant is neither responsible for its genetics nor its environment and nurturance as a child. This is perhaps the single most important inference I wish to make, and leads to my third point.

My third principle - and maybe the hardest for all of us to remember - is this: *don't blame the victim*!

Even if the victim is you. Even if you are full of guilt and shame and keep saying, "Yes, but maybe I should have/could have done/not done this or that." Children of divorce do this to themselves too. It still doesn't make them responsible for their parents' separation.

I realize there are spiritual theories and explanations here, and while I bow to them, I cannot present and encompass them all. However I would point out, to anyone who is taught that we 'choose' our circumstances, that this is not a conscious process. The persons living with the 'chosen' handicap suffer just as much as if it had been imposed on them from the outside. Thus, in this sense they are still a victim of forces they could not control.

There is a recent trend in our society to make 'victim' a dirty word. Granted we all are capable of choosing our response to every circumstance; yet if one did not choose the circumstance knowingly, I think the word 'victim' is appropriate. It does not lessen the person who has been harmed, merely indicates that the initiating party was someone other. That is the sense in which I apply the word.

Myths take a long time to die. There is still plenty of stigma, blame, and shame involved in being mentally ill (people who suffer from other chronic or 'invisible' illnesses have much the same problem). There's very little validation. Certain religions may try to tell us that if we only had enough faith, we would be healed. Certain friends may tell us that we just don't try hard enough. Relatives and self-help programs may imply that we should merely 'control ourselves.' It's hard to keep believing, in the face of the untutored but strident majority, that our illness is as legitimate and deserves as much gentleness and care as any other major health problem.

Our shame is not necessary.

Yes, our symptoms may put us in painful or embarrassing situations. They can change, limit, and fracture our lives. And yes, sometimes we will hurt those around us and they will be angry. A lot of rejection and loneliness can come with the territory. All of this makes life rough.

But it does not make you a bad person!

Graham Nelson, a banker and novelist from the U.K., puts it this way: "You know how some people catch a nasty flu? Well, that's all this is – it's not your fault, it's an illness and in time, you WILL feel better."

Those with special chemistry can no more be blamed for their symptoms than a horse with a broken leg can be blamed for limping.

Lastly, my most important assumption is that you don't have to believe my assumptions. My experience shows that the Twelve Steps work if one applies them diligently, no matter what one may privately think about the 'causes' of this or that. They are simply effective.

An Acronym for Us

I'd like to propose a term a little less cumbersome than 'The Mentally Ill.' That covers so much ground! And it is such a mouthful. It also puts us firmly in the 'sick' category, which may not be desirable.

What do all these psychiatric conditions, all these types of abnormal psychology, have in common? My answer: altered states.

There is really not much happening in an abnormal psyche that does not happen in a 'normal' brain under certain circumstances. We are all capable of every kind of human emotion and reaction, even the most extreme and scary. Most people have 'heard voices' – the little one that reminds them they left their gloves on the table, or the one that makes them turn and ask, "What did you say?" when no one has said anything. We experience an altered state every night during sleep. Athletes talk about reaching 'The Zone' – an endorphin-induced altered state that is quite common and in no way frightening or illegal. There are many other examples in everyday life, if you think about it.

It is just that some of us are able to reach these states arbitrarily, at an extreme, when there seems to be no stimulus in the environment.

What do I mean? Well, let me put it this way. In my twenties I did some mild experimentation with recreational drugs at parties. I found there were certain effects I already could reach on my own without pills, and I didn't want them. Speed was a lot like Mania (though I didn't call it that at the time). Downers and Depression had a lot in common. Paranoia I could reach all by myself without marijuana, thank you very much.

I was *Prone to Altered States of Consciousness*, without any help from outside. Anxiety, Panic, the mental place from which we hear voices, the heightened awareness and terror of a Panic Attack, etc., these are all altered states. We get them for free.

A word here about their nature: altered states are not all strange or even bad. Some of them can be extremely appropriate, depending on your culture, religion, or situation. I regularly use them to produce poetry[4]; indeed, the delicious altered state accompanying good writing is one of the reasons some of us love to do it so much. Certain religions and rituals may have altered states as their goals – and I am not only talking about Native American Indians or tribal Shamans here, but some well-established Christian churches. What, after all, is all that ritual chanting and music and incense *for*, if not to induce a receptive, slightly hypnotic state of mind? Sometimes visions or a voice of guidance is *desired* and *praised*, as in the case of certain saints and their visions. Furthermore, meditation is an altered state that is entered into purposely to take us to places we cannot reach with the rational mind. It is said by some experts – and I believe them – that drugs pose a problem for people partly because they take a person to places that only years of meditation can prepare one for. Others are not ready, and the effect on them can be catastrophic.

On the other hand, some religions *require* the enhancement of experience by use of certain potent plants or drugs, and this cannot realistically be considered abuse, even if use is heavy and regular. (Abuse can only be defined as that amount of usage which makes a person's ordinary life fall apart while at the same time s/he is unable to stop using despite these results.) Many people have forgotten, too, that the original goal of the sixties' drug experimentation was precisely to *expand one's perception* and reach new states of mind. It was only in the later, broader culture that it became a recreational amusement, a hit at parties, and a problem. And some people, loosely called New Age, have found that these states can be of positive worth

---

[4] Some of us lose the ability to reach desired altered states when we take our medications. This is NOT a good excuse to stop medications. You will find, as I have, that these mental 'places' are still available to you…it just may be harder to get there, and take some conscious work. I take long walks, listen to music, and stare into fires, for instance.

and meaning, used for the betterment of the world and spiritual advancement.

The challenge – and the unmanageability - comes in when these altered states are *unwanted*, when they come upon you randomly, uncontrollably, at moments when you need rational, day-to-day consciousness; or when you are not *aware* that you are in an altered state, and believe your reality is the same as everyone else's.

To recap: I am not claiming that altered states are real or imaginary, good or evil, physical or spiritual. You will surely come to your own conclusions about this. I am merely pointing out that they are human, and that some folks experience them much more often.

So what I would say that what we 'mentally ill' have in common is that we are **Prone to Altered States of Consciousness: PASC**. It is not a deprecating term. It is merely descriptive.

I will be using that term for easy reference. I hope you will find it useful - both easier to say and a bit more accurate than phrases like 'psychiatric condition.'

Or you can take a tip from the creators of 'special needs' and say we have 'special chemistry.' It's a little PC for my taste, but it's useful shorthand.

Why the Twelve Steps

What are they, anyway?

Some of you know the Twelve Steps is a program of change that was originally developed to help alcoholics overcome their addiction. It is fairly simple, and just what it sounds like: Twelve Steps of decision and/or action that help you repair and change your life. They do not make the problem go away. They allow us to somehow *bypass* it, or work with it, by the use of spiritual and psychological principles.

The Steps have been so successful over the years that they have been applied to everything from overeating to picking your nose. It's kind of been overdone. But do they apply to the PASC? I have used them, and I say 'yes.'

Some of us are stuck to our old ways, and we only want to use the Steps for addiction, even though we have other problems.

Those who have an addiction plus a mental disorder are part of what is known as the dual diagnosis population.

For simplicity's sake, I'm going to assume that the dual-diagnosis members of my audience are already working to solve their substance abuse. There are plenty of good new books out on the subject, and the original Twelve-Step Groups are geared for them.

It is the dually-diagnosed whom I wish to address for a moment (whoever else may be listening in).

Those of us with dual diagnoses tend to get lost in the Anonymous crowd. We are the recovering, the hardworking, the grateful -- and the lonely. We are the ones who did all our footwork, but still didn't get better. We are the weird among the weird. We don't feel welcome. We don't speak up. And we need to.

When you've got this kind of double-whammy, you can't help wondering about your value. Did I do something horribly wrong? Am I being punished for sins I committed in a previous life? Am I simply a weak personality? Is it just bad DNA? Can we posit that, in trying to get away from the exquisite misery of our illnesses, some of us adopted alcohol, drugs, and other self-destructive behaviors just for relief? Is the electrical brain mis-wiring so similar that the conditions develop in tandem?

The temptation is to shove these questions back in the closet. I know. I did it for eight years. It's hard enough keeping things together as it is, right? I've already worked a program, you say. I've done good. I don't drink (overeat, shoot-up, whatever - you fill in the blank) any more. Besides, what on earth does mental illness have to do with Anonymous meetings?

Can't I quit now? Haven't I done enough?

Yes, you have. Nobody can or should push anybody into another new program. To paraphrase Melody Beattie, author of <u>Codependent No More,</u> one big problem ought to be enough in one lifetime. If life were fair, that's how it would be.

What I am suggesting has nothing to do with how good we are or how hard we've tried. What I am suggesting is that we expand our Twelve-Step efforts to include our special chemistry *because it will make us feel better*. And we *deserve* to feel better!

More Will Be Revealed

This phrase is used constantly among Twelve-Step Members. It means the further you go into this work, the more you'll find out. It's never all visible at the start.

The first three Steps help us shed the immense burden of shame and blame we place on ourselves for the symptoms we can't change. They may even help our symptoms in some cases, simply because of the removal of some of that enormous emotional stress.

Certain responsibilities and repair are still required of us, though, particularly if our symptoms tend to jump out and attack other people. The Fourth through Ninth Steps help us with this. They also help us separate our *selves* from our *chemistry*, and deal with the resentment we feel toward those who stereotype and hurt us.

From the Tenth Step on, we get to start having our meaningful lives back, not by a magical cure but by means of clear vision and spiritual sanity. Spiritual sanity is what it's all about. Lest you balk at the word 'spiritual', I'm really just talking about inner peace, or balance.

Please notice: there are many indigenous religions in which insanity and spirituality are not thought of as polar opposites. There is a tendency for people of the Big Three religions to regard 'wholeness' as equal to clinical definitions of 'mental health.' But many subcultures accept that spiritually whole people can come from the ranks of the PASC. The mind is seen as almost another form of 'body,' which is subject to illness; and whether or not one has a healthy mind, one is still capable of having a healthy spirit.

Sharing is the other thing it's all about. As in any form of Twelve-Step program, sharing what we have is critical.

Becoming spiritually sane is not a selfish act. Not only do we need the program, but the program needs us. Through our unique and hard-won insights, we have much to offer.

I believe that applying the Twelve Steps to my condition has increased my functional sanity. I know for certain it makes the nonfunctional days easier to take. And I feel that, for the first time since my diagnosis, I am beginning to have something to give back to the world. I can see beyond the chain-link fence of insanity, and the power I used to waste on self-blame can now be used for better things.

It may not work for you exactly the same way it worked for me. But as my detox counselor used to say, "Try it. If you don't like it, at the end of thirty days, we will cheerfully refund your misery in full."

If you are tired of the misery and isolation, if the doctors and pills by themselves just aren't fixing things, if you are willing to go to any lengths to acquire inner peace, it's time to start with Step One.

WE, THE INVISIBLE

Steps One to Three

"Yesterday, upon the stair,
I met a man who wasn't there.
He wasn't there again today.
I wish that man would go away!"
-- William Hughes Mearns

STEP ONE

Admit Your Condition

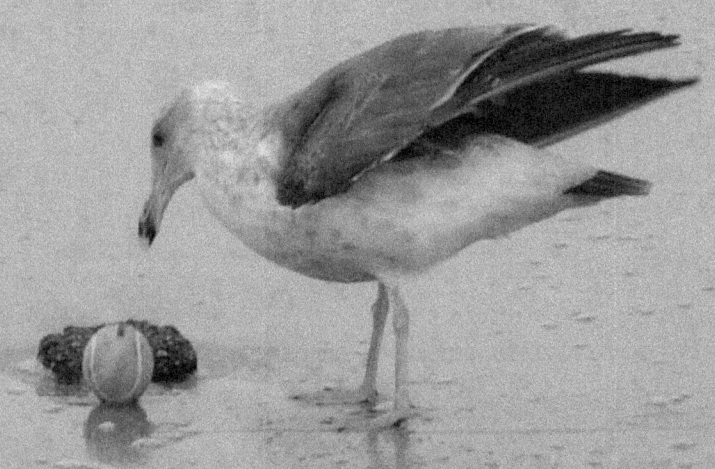

"We admitted we were powerless
over mental illness,
and that our lives had become unmanageable."
--adapted from the Twelve Steps
of AA

Step One

The executive director of the Center for Independent Living in Berkeley, California, once gave a workshop about the Americans with Disabilities Act. In the course of the workshop, he asked his audience to guess how many forms of disabilities there were. None of us guessed right. There are nine hundred.

Nine hundred.

So it might seem arrogant to say that the mentally ill feel a greater need of control than any other group. But it's true.

Every disability involves loss of control over some area of one's body or one's life. Usually both. The blind, the deaf, diabetics, stroke victims, amputees, epileptics, paraplegics and quadriplegics - all of these people and hundreds of others know the bitterness of loss of control and heightened dependency on others.

But at least they get to think their own thoughts!

To have no power over your own mind is the bitterest betrayal of all.

So we don't have control, and we crave it. And the first Step, which might look obvious and easy to outsiders, can often turn into a wrestling match between us and our basic human dignity.

Admitting you are not in control of your brain may be the single hardest thing you will ever do. That is why this chapter is the longest in the book.

It reminds me of a joke that was current in psychological circles about 10 years ago: *The truth will set you free, but first it will make you miserable.*

Don't kid yourself. Mental illness is not for sissies.

Beyond the primitive fear of that murky term 'madness', we have a realistic fear of what happens *next*. Will I lose my job? Then how will I support myself? Will I end up on welfare? Will my friends reject me? What will they think of me now? What do I think of myself? Will I end up in 'the loony bin'? Will I lose my mind entirely? What happens then?

Next to facing all that, making sense of the rest of life with special chemistry is just a matter of logistics.

Nobody wants to cop to a condition that may make them into a dependant. Eddie Smith, a security guard, has been facing these issues all his life. He had hallucinations as a child, and was written up by teachers as having various phobias and difficulties all through primary school. At the age of 19, he was involved in a motor-scooter accident that nearly took off his leg. For weeks he stayed in the hospital while doctors debated whether the limb could be saved or needed amputation. And he developed his first concrete diagnosis.

> "So I explained to the doctor – not as a feeling but as a fact – 'Here's my problem. God has positioned another truck in the parking lot of this hospital. And the plan is that on the day that I'm released, that truck will run me over again, finally killing me. And I can't see that truck now but I know it's there'.
>
> "And he said, 'Well, you are Paranoid.'"

Big horse pills followed, and toward the end of the stay Eddie was willing to allow that maybe the truck was not actually there.

At 23 he had another breakdown and drove himself to a nearby Southern California hospital. They decided he was a 'borderline psychotic' and let him drive himself home the same day, after administering Thorazine – a dangerous maneuver that would not be tolerated today. And he went straight back to full-time college and a job and family life.

Later, after another breakdown in San Francisco, he was tagged with Atypical Depression and actually admitted to the hospital for three weeks – a first. Shortly after leaving he became so anxious he sought an emergency clinic again and was put in a padded room. They talked him over among themselves, gave him some Valium, and sent him home with a vague label of 'some kind of Anxiety Disorder.'

When I asked him which diagnosis he felt was correct, he said all of them were.

> "Clearly I saw that the Paranoia diagnosis was true. So that was fine. Borderline Psychosis was obviously true. Atypical Depression was true; they were just giving me the wrong medicines. And the major failing this whole time was that they didn't diagnose Anxiety Disorder.

> "I knew I was crazy. The diagnosis for some people is like an insult. Whereas I'm amazed I'm not at Napa [a center for the dangerously insane]. So whatever you have to add is not going to blow my mind."

Eddie continued to work at a number of low-paying jobs all through his forties, ending as a security guard. Holding a job was difficult for him. I believe at one time he told me he had held 78 positions. His great fear, like many of us, was that he would become totally dependent. And not everybody has someone who will support them in such disability.

> "I was saying to my most recent therapist – she was saying, 'Well, you have friends, right?' I said, 'Yes, I do. But there's a little problem. Since they're all as crazy as me or way crazier, then it's sort of the drowning trying to cling to other drowning people to get saved. It's not like there's one of them that can say, 'I'm healthy. And what we'll do here is we'll give you a job and we'll allow it to be flexible'; or 'You'll stay in our cottage in the

back of our mansion, and that's how we'll
solve it'; or a family member saying, 'What
we'll do is we'll take the old study and convert
it into your room and you'll just have to grow
old with us.'

"I've seen that happen many times. I
have a friend who passed away many years
ago, for whom the final plan was, he lived at
Mom's house, forever. And it's very, very
common. So, for instance, in the [poor]
community, those people live with Mom
forever.

"...There's more belief in *unconditional*
love. I may be a horrible parent and don't
know what to do. And that may be part of the
reason he went insane. Nonetheless, in my
mind, I just believe that you do this, forever.
Which doesn't really exist in the [wealthier]
culture any more."

We are afraid of admitting to a condition that may
change everything else in our lives. It is hardest the first time we
face it squarely, when all the possible dangers are unknown. But
facing such problems – and solving them – is something any
person with chronic illness is familiar with. Coming to
permanent terms with our special chemistry, and the limitations
it may impose, can be a lifelong task. Acceptance and non-
acceptance tend to come in waves, following a cycle all their
own.

After you've faced facts, the rest is arrangements and
fallbacks. The remainder of this book will help you with that.

Lisa, the Alabama mother we encountered before, had
trouble accepting her diagnosis, too:

"I was previously diagnosed with
chronic anxiety in my early 20's. Many years

later, and less than two years ago, a neurologist diagnosed me as Bipolar. I was angry, and I argued with him, but he stood his ground and prescribed the medications... Now, after taking the medications and researching the condition, I realize he was right, and I'm thankful someone finally offered me the help I so desperately needed."

If you've suspected that 'something is wrong,' you may be happy to have a name for it at last. Once it has a name, it has a course of treatment. For me, it was like a light going on in a dark room.

Jessica, an auburn-haired graduate student in psychology, actually found her diagnosis a relief. Like many PASC, she has a grab bag of disorders: Generalized Anxiety Disorder, adult ADHD, and what she describes as 'some kind of Depression' that does not totally incapacitate her (possibly Dysthymia?).

"It helped to get some idea of what it was, you know. Or, to figure out that what I call 'my hysterical freak-outs' were actually something involving Anxiety Disorder helped, because I had much worse names for it."

The discovery that you are PASC can be very dramatic and disturbing.

Vivien, a curvaceous single mother, had a sudden descent into Schizo-affective Disorder in her twenties. She was taking guitar lessons and had a private crush on her teacher. She used to wonder whether he returned her interest or not. Then one strange night she started hearing voices in her head. The voices told her that her teacher was secretly in love with her and wanted her to come and find him. They even told her that he was suicidal and needed her desperately.

So she wandered the gritty Mission District of San Francisco late at night, trying random doors of strange apartments. People called in and reported her, and eventually police picked her up. She says it started this way:

> "I felt I was dying, myself. Because...I went back to my old apartment, and I tested the handle of my apartment door, and I heard a word. And what I heard was like 'Hell, hell, hell, hell.'"

> "I touched the apartment doorknob. And it was like I had an electric shock, touching the knob of the door. And so I went and tried to find my guitar teacher, and heard words [in my head] like, 'Go to Studio [so-and-so], you'll find him there.' And so I got on the bus and I went."

Her sister had to forcibly detain her in the apartment the next night to keep it from happening again. Soon she was living on her parents' couch, unable to work. Nevertheless, when she was given her diagnosis, she didn't think she needed any medication. In the end it was her parents who insisted. It is not unusual for people in even the worst condition to think that having a label and a little therapy is enough.

But all you have to do is look at their subsequent behavior to see that they are fooling themselves. Vivien was unable to work at her skilled job as a silk screener even after months of medical leave. Something in her brain had checked out for good.

> "It changed me that I forgot some things," she says. "I forgot how to run my machine. It had fried my brain, and I would think about being in front of the machine and trying to run it and not be able to run it."

All of this waffling about one's condition is normal, and excusable. But it stands directly in the way of 'admitting our powerlessness,' which is the whole point of the First Step.

If you don't admit you're powerless, you can't get help.

Many people find accepting their diagnosis to be the hardest part. For others, it is having to take the pills.

Shanna, the only teenager among my interviewees, says that it was her anger and Depressions that first clued her in to what was wrong.

"Okay, when I get Depressed, it comes for no apparent reason. It comes from reasons, but reasons that shouldn't matter any more. There can be reasons but they're so small...Like, even if I just look at my brother and sisters, I just have to go to my room and cry. Like I'll just pick on them and stuff, and then I'll say, 'wow, I'm so mean to them,' and I'll just go to my room and cry.

"One of my biggest fears of my whole entire life was having my Dad die. There's times like this Christmas, I had to go...I just had to go to the bathroom for probably about 30, 45 minutes, and cry and cry, I just couldn't stand it, I'd look at Daddy and I couldn't stand it. It was so random, though. My boyfriend was here, and he's, like, knocking on the door going 'What's wrong, what's wrong?' And I said, 'I can't come out. If I come out right now, it's just going to get worse.'

"Probably the thing that was most noticeable to me was my anger. By the time I was eleven, I was having self-mutilation and stuff. I was always hitting things and stuff like that, because I had no other way to cope with it...and I didn't know if Mama would judge me or not.

"I had early symptoms, but we didn't

know they were early symptoms until I put my
hand through the wall...We had gotten in a
little fight...I went outside and I hit something,
and my knuckles were messed up. I came
inside, and I decided I had to tell her, right? I
told her. And she was just, like, 'Well we're
going to have to take you to the doctor,
because this could be something.'"

What Shanna did not know was that her mother was
Bipolar and under treatment already.

"The day that she told me she was Bipolar
was the first day I ever really talked to her...
she'd been through it. But I had no idea. All
that stuff that I had seen Mom do, or heard my
Mom do? It made sense, then.

"When Momma found out, we went to the
doctor, a regular family doctor. And he put me
on Zoloft. I hated it. I could not stand it. It
made me more Depressed. They told me I
needed to go see the Mental Health Center.

"I told Momma, 'I'm not going.' I told her
that they were just going to lock me up.
Because I knew if I went, they would find out –
at the time all that was hidden, that I was all
cutting [myself] and everything, and Momma
didn't know about that yet. But the reason I
didn't want to go to Mental Health Center was
because I thought if I did, that that was going
to come out."

I think Shanna's account touches on a deep fear held by
most of us: "They were just going to lock me up." She says the
same thing about her public school: "I don't want to go to
public 'cause I don't want to freak a teacher out and make her

send me to a mental institution or something." And once she was undergoing counseling, she felt as if the possibility was being held over her head.

> "The looks they give you when you tell them things. That drives me up the wall...I'll tell them something and they'll give me this look, like,' You better watch what you say or I'll send you somewhere.' That makes me mad. Or like the fear you have when you walk in. Or the fear you have when you say something. Because even though I don't go there hardly any more – when I have refills, I do – but when I do go, I'm pretty much like, if I say something I better sugar-coat this, so that they don't send me to...I know the mental institution is not – the mental hospital isn't that bad of a place, but –

> "I'm not judging anybody who has been. I just have a fear of going, because I've never been. It's like they're threatening you with it, pretty much. They want that over your head. I don't know...Um. I mean, if I need to go, I will go. But if somebody *makes* me go – my mindset, when I get out, they'll – they won't be happy!"

Folks, I have news. The psychiatric wing of the average hospital is a very boring place. Not much happens there. I've been, many times, and fear is just about my *last* reaction.

The problem is, we have all been exposed to the Boogie Man of "Bedlam," the horrible place where they used to lock up inmates, abuse them, and show stylish visitors around for a price, as if the PASC were animals in the zoo. We have heard too about the "treatments" offered in earlier centuries, some of which were torturous. And we have seen too many dramatic and scary scenes in books and movies.

The modern psychiatric wing is just a safe place to stay

while you get it together. I have been there somewhere between five and seven times. It was so dull, I can't really remember the exact number.

The trick is to go in under your own steam. Then, there are no white-coated attendants, police, or straitjackets. You just call your doctor, and tell him/her you need to be hospitalized. Once the doctor is satisfied, through questioning, that you need to go, then s/he arranges everything, and you just get someone to drive you there, and show up at the agreed time.

They check you in, which is tedious and involves a lot of paper-signing about your rights and responsibilities – the fruit of modern reform laws. You are not signing away your freedom. You are perfectly free to leave at any time. They just want to make sure you understand exactly what you are doing. Nobody is going to forcibly detain you. It's harder to get *in* these days than get *out*.

In fact, the problem with hospital stays in modern America is that they are often too short. Patients' insurance simply will not cover them for very long, and someone who could use a month of protection and rest will probably get only 10 to 14 days. Even outpatient care can be truncated. I once knew a man, still quite suicidal, who was told he was being discharged from day treatment. The reason? He had taken a shower and shaved. This was 'improvement' enough to try and dismiss him. Apparently they were not happy with his insurance plan. Maybe health care reform will change this.

Once you've signed all the papers, you have to do the one 'degrading' thing, which is give up anything on your person that could possibly be harmful. Yes, even your fingernail clippers and shaving things. They will be re-issued to you when you need them, and put away behind the nurses' desk afterwards. This may make you feel a little silly and kindergarten-ish. But you know and I know that they will be the first ones to be blamed if someone manages to hang themselves by their shoelaces.

Despair is not very discriminating. In protecting themselves, they are protecting you.

You usually have to give up your cigarettes as well – which I understand is part of hospital hygiene, but is a very bad idea for people who are under far too much stress to begin with. The PASC often tend to be heavy smokers. Hospital time is just when you need your crutches the most. If you are lucky, there may be a little room somewhere in which patients who smoke are allowed to gather once or twice a day. Most places do not have this amenity, however.

And that's about it. You'll probably have a single bed in a room with a few others – no, they will not be maniacs with wild eyes who need to be restrained every day, though they may have some odd ideas – and for the first few days you may have lots of blood tests and such so they can see how you are doing physically. There will be regular mealtimes which will probably exclude caffeine of any kind, and there will be regular group therapy. The therapy is generally not brilliant, as nobody in the group is in very good shape; but some is better than none. There'll be a sort of living room somewhere with a TV and whatever other entertainment may be provided – usually paperbacks of the drugstore variety – and possibly an exercise room with a piece of equipment or two. You can see visitors during certain hours, and your visitors can bring you anything within the safety rules. Your doctor, or a staff doctor, will visit you at regular intervals. Nurses will bring you your medicine at the appointed times.

It's really very dull. Just a safe place to be taken care of until you are ready to face things again. Nothing scary, and nothing exciting. All the real action is going on in your mind!

Of course, if you refuse to go in until they come and take you away, it's going to be more dramatic than that. I would advise going in under your own power. It can be messy and expensive and embarrassing to be carried off. Much better to say you need a leave of absence and just disappear from work for a week or two. The hospital is generally not allowed to even confirm to callers whether you are a patient there or not, so it can be your secret.

Not only did Shanna worry about being hospitalized, like many people she did not want to take medicine – even after she could see that it was helping.

"I'm not as judgmental, not as angry. I've

calmed down a lot...I'm reacting, but not as intensely...I'm still angry, but I can cope with it, in my head. I don't have to do bad things to cope with it.

"I told Mom that I didn't need medicine, and if they put me on medicine – I was terrified of medicine. Because I didn't want to alter myself, even though I knew I needed it. I had been that way for so long that I got used to it, and I was fine with it.

"Now that I've been on medicine, I kind of see where it is better, but I pray one day I'll get taken off of it, and I'll be fine. Only I don't really see it happening. Because I'm extremely Bipolar without my medicine. Right. Like, [if] I'm off my medicine pretty much, and if I'm having to wait for refills or something – even if I'm off for a day, though it's still in my system, it just alters me.

"Momma, I was talking to her the other day, I was like, 'Am I ready to be taken off medicines?' Because I've got a thing about not wanting to be on medicines. And she's like, 'I'd rather you didn't.'"

There are people who refuse, and there are people who go on and off their medicines when it suits them. Doctors call this 'non-compliance,' an unhelpful term that makes us sound like naughty school children. But non-compliance is a serious problem; it can get us and everybody we love in a lot of trouble. I'll talk about this in more detail in the section 'Outer Tips for Inner Peace.'

The point is, nobody likes having a psychiatric label. Even if we accept the label, we often don't want to take the next steps. But it is the only way to get our lives into any kind of usable shape. Admitting your condition is the heart of the First

Step. And I know just how hard it is.

I kind of had to have my diagnosis shoved down my throat. One day, long after my diagnosis and refusal of medicine, I was walking on the beach. I had been worrying, something I did well and often. I was walking along Ocean Beach in San Francisco on a cold, blustery day, and I was feeling terrible anxiety about my future.

It had never occurred to me before that I did not have much of a future. I was a mid-level clerk in a bank, and had no college degree or math aptitude. I had grand plans of traveling Europe, going to Venice for a honeymoon, writing books without keeping an ordinary job, living in a house with multiple wings, and hiring a nanny to take care of any children! Yet the truth was, I lived in a basement and couldn't keep up with my charge cards. So suddenly, that day, I started counting up the cost of my dreams – and realized that I didn't stand a chance.

Well, what can I say to describe this? I panicked in a rising, spiraling, obsessive way that had nothing to do with sanity. I was holding myself against the wind; I was pounding my arms against myself, and pacing up and down. And suddenly I heard a voice inside my head telling me that if I went home RIGHT NOW, without stopping, I would get a miracle phone call that would solve all my problems.

I argued with this voice, telling it silly things like "I HAVE to stop on the way home, because I am out of cigarettes!" (I was a heavy drinker and smoker at the time.) The voice said, "Then you will miss The Call." And I really didn't quite know what to think. My logic said 'No,' but my childhood training told me that God could talk to anyone, and you never knew what He might say. I argued this back and forth in my head for a long time.

At length, I kind of glanced up and realized that everyone on the beach was avoiding me. I saw that I was pacing up and down talking to myself in a shaky high voice, beating my arms.

I thought, "If I were them – if I didn't know better – I'd think I was crazy."

And then I got it.

I *was* crazy.

I really was.

This was what crazy looked like. This was what crazy felt like. This was me.

I drove home (stopping for cigarettes!) and called my therapist. "You know those pills you talked about? I think I need them." She hooked me up with a psychiatrist, and my long slow healing began.

I had to *see* myself. And I had to do that by myself. No one else can tell you.

The First Step asks us to admit that we are powerless. Why? Because there is *no* other way to begin to get better.

But society makes 'mental illness' so scary that it's very hard to do this.

The fact that some people *blame* us for our illness doesn't help much. If they just said, 'Oh, you're ill, let's help you,' perhaps we would not be so afraid.

There is a certain kind of guilt that the PASC carry around. Maybe, for Americans, it's our Calvinist heritage. If you're ill, does it mean you're not one of God's Chosen? Maybe it's the years and years before diagnosis, when people kept criticizing us and staring at us and saying, "What is wrong with you? Snap out of it!" We're told we're over-sensitive, and ought to take things more lightly, or that we're rude or selfish or bitchy. Maybe they said we were bad-tempered and ungrateful. Maybe they suggested that we join a therapy group, do affirmations, play tennis to work up a sweat and use that energy, eat lots of chicken soup...whatever. Maybe we tried some (or all) of these things (or maybe we told them to go to hell). But at some point, the message got through anyway: *It is all your fault! You could be better, if you really tried.*

Gabriel, a newly married graduate student, describes his situation this way:

> "It's hard having an illness that defies logic...I'd like to say, 'A led to B led to C,' but it's not that simple. I have a disease. It causes my thinking to deviate wildly...but there's no cause and effect other than my illness...'That's

a cop-out' some say. 'Take responsibility for your actions.'

"My loved ones, my fiancée, friends and family all deserve some sort of explanation for the heartache, stress and worry I've caused. It's frustrating not to be able to offer it."

Shanna says, "A lot of people, it's not that they don't care, they just don't have enough determination to make it all the way there."

Sick from the Start

Of course, some of us have never been 'normal' in the first place. We don't know what that's like.

I became Bipolar at 13 years old, with the onset of puberty. And that's all I thought it was. That's all anybody around me thought, too. I was a 'drama queen.' I was 'difficult.' I was 'volatile.' All I knew was that I was miserable, always.

At first I thought it was my family's fault. After all, they were strict authoritarian fundamentalists and I was a born bohemian. Not a good match. I thought that when I left home, all would be well. But when I left home, there was reality – and poverty. And then there were some very ill-chosen friends and boyfriends, and a job I hated. It wasn't until I had a two-year relationship with a very loving, giving man – *and felt just the same* – that I finally saw that the problem was in me. I was 26 before my Bipolar condition was discovered. I was 34 before I first experienced a quiet mind that allowed me to think in peace. So when did I get a chance to 'just try harder'? I had no idea *what* adult sanity *felt like*. I was a child, and then I was insane. There was nothing in between.

Sally, a painter and post-graduate student in spiritual studies, became symptomatic at 13 as well:

"I had a breakdown at thirteen out of the blue. However, the pervious year, I did go through a Depression all year. At the time, I felt it was a spiritual experience. I was into the Bible at the time, and I thought that things like my breakdown must've happened in the Bible all the time.

      "...My father did start hating me after I was diagnosed. I moved out at fifteen. We all went to family therapy."

How is a 13 year old supposed to assess her sanity and rebuild her family? *If you don't have a benchmark of what 'sane' is, how can you tell when you're not?*
    You remember Eddie Smith? He had his first delusions at age five.

      "...Because my parents were in such denial, I don't know what the diagnosis was, but I was medicated as a five-year-old. And I did hallucinate.

      "...I hallucinated that there was a man in my room. So, I was lonely and crying out, and I saw a man that I thought was my dad come in the room and watch over me. Silently.

      "I went, 'Dad, dad,' but there was no answer. I said, 'Dad, what are you doing?' Ran up, touched him – he was like stone...Ran back to my bed. 'Who are you?' And then, the door opened, he silently left.

      "The next day, I'm like, 'Dad, how come you came to my room last night and stood there but you wouldn't talk to me?' They're like, 'We didn't hear you call out. We didn't come to your room.'

"…And then, I'd be laying [sic] in bed, and on different nights, even God (or the devil) would go, '…we want you…come to us' in this whispering voice. And so I was having audio hallucinations. Now those, I couldn't even say my parents played a trick on me, because there was no vision of my parents or their voice or anything. It was just God in the wall, or the devil some nights in the wall; and me saying, 'No, I don't want to go with you!'"

It's hard to imagine how a five-year-old could have 'just tried harder' to be a little more sane and normal.

Jessica remembers trouble starting in kindergarten:

"I've always had some kind of problem. Even before I was diagnosed.

"I went through kindergarten and I wasn't behaving like the other kids. I would hide in the coat closet. Because they wanted me to go play with the dolls, but the other girls didn't *want* me to play with the dolls, because I was too rough and they would throw me out of the dollhouse. But if I tried to go play with the boys and the trucks, they wouldn't let me do that because I was a girl. So I just would hide in the coat closet. And I would do other things that disrupted the class, so I was in the Principal's office almost every day. The school told my parents I had to go and get psychological testing.

"So then they said I had minimal brain dysfunction, which meant they couldn't find anything wrong, but there had to be something wrong or I wouldn't be acting that way. I had to have some kind of minimal brain damage or something…which was probably ADHD.

"…there's really no 'before' for me."

Shelley Scirocco, a slim, blonde, high-energy Bipolar painter, says her very first memory is of a psychotic break:

"I went completely ballistic in a store. My mother said I went completely – and I was tearing things, and they had the security people – she said she was so scared….I was angry. I was afraid. There was fear – and rage…It was the first thing I ever remember doing in my life. They say the first thing you *consciously* remember, you will enact that, over and over again. I have had that – haven't I? Haven't I been a little messy, bad wind blowing around?"

Yet she was not sent to a doctor until she was in her teens, and not correctly diagnosed until she was 28.

"I was between 14 and 15, and they didn't know, really, what was wrong. They just said, 'You have a really hyperactive child'… Well, they did that when I was young. Then they didn't give me any medicine. They just said, 'No, she's all right; she's a real hyper kid. She's a very creative child, you know that. Look at her!'….My parents just said, 'No, she's not [sick], she's just a musician. She's an artist. There's nothing wrong with her at all.' They were in denial. Denial. My parents were.

"I kept going back intermittently to psychiatrists. Just, like, when they could afford

it or whatever. I don't know what the reason
was. I don't.

"...so after [college] it just sort of
became like, man, I'm Depressed. Goddamn,
I'm Depressed! I've got to do something. So I
went to Massachusetts, I got in this band --
Manically doing things, you know, like
Maniacally, you know. Manic-Depressives
travel a lot! They like to travel, they like to
shop, they like to move...I had a LOT of
energy, boy, I slept 4 hours a night! I was never
sleeping. Never. I was always up, I was Manic.
And I was always going somewhere.

"I didn't get diagnosed officially till I
was 28. Because I was out HERE, and I said,
'There's something wrooong with me.' That's
what I said. To myself...So I went to this place
and they said, 'You're Manic-Depressive.
You're a classic Manic-Depressive.' I went,
'ahhhh...relief!' That made a lot of sense."

But Americans are obsessed with perfection, and
transcending impossible obstacles.[1] We revel in stories of rags to
riches, of the great marathon runner who suffered from polio in
childhood, of the quadriplegic who paints with a brush in her
teeth. The burden of bearing up, of overcoming everything with
swashbuckling style, is enough to make any ordinary mortal
feel inadequate.

For those of us whose dysfunction is invisible, shame is a
natural companion. And it is crushing. It can make us slink off

---

[1] In other cultures and times, there is often a greater acknowledgement of the hand of
fate, whether it be the flow of the universe in Taoism, or the will of the gods in
Hinduism (a concept also shared by the ancient Romans). A person with PASC can
be treated with more empathy in times and places where our own lack of control is
better understood.

to dark corners with our tails tucked, hide out in jobs for which we're overqualified, stay in stifling relationships because we believe no one else will have us.

After all, how can you help feeling like a loser when your best friend just dropped you because you did something you can't remember? Or you have to call someone to bring you home from the local hospital, after being picked up by the police? Or you wake up running naked down Main Street at midnight? Or you just silenced an entire room by something that sort of fell out of your mouth when you weren't looking? Or you discover that some part of you went out shopping and charged $30,000 worth of nonrefundable merchandise?

These things are hard to live with, and they make us feel shame. We feel we 'should' be able to control them.

Gabriel recounts:

> "When I relapsed I maxed out three credit cards and had no choice but to declare bankruptcy, which comes with consequences of its own. When it's time for a bigger house in the next few years, it'll have to be in her name. Same for a car, or anything else that requires a credit check. In the moment when I put that engagement ring on her finger, she wasn't thinking of all that. But now it's staring us in the face, and I struggle to come to terms with the results of all the ill-advised actions I've taken. I can give my personal guarantee that the events of last summer won't repeat themselves, but from her point of view, what's that really worth? I haven't done much to earn a lot of trust and faith. Ironically, those things are exactly what I need right now."

Of course we feel rotten! And the temptation to isolate, to skulk around and stop having a life, is sometimes irresistible. As Gabriel puts it:

"Sometimes I feel as though I'm buried.
On the bleakest days, I simply remind myself
to eat, sleep, bathe, and do the maintenance
that will get me through to a better day."

In a way, coming to PASC via a substance abuse program
is even worse. Because you do all your homework, but you still
don't 'get well.' After all, isn't this the place where the weird get
better? Isn't this supposed to save us?[2] Isn't this the one place
where everybody can belong and be OK? But week after month
after year goes by. And maybe we do get better — some. Maybe
the compulsion to drink does lift, and our lives gets back on
track — partly.

But we are still having Manic episodes or hallucinations
or Panic Attacks or what-have-you; and our relationships still
suck; and we still have to lie to our bosses about the real reason
we couldn't work last Tuesday. Maybe we can't get any 'clean'
time because we relapse during episodes (the Bipolar, for
instance, are 30% more likely to become alcoholics than the
'normal' population - did anyone tell you that?). It is my
personal theory that substance abuse is one of the commoner
reactions to special chemistry.

We start to think that, after all, maybe it IS just us. Maybe
we're just too defective, too lazy, too stupid, too degenerate, too
undisciplined.

First of all, it's not true.

Secondly, there is a trick built into this blaming and
shaming business, and as long as you stick to those attitudes,
emotional recovery can't happen.

---

[2] In monotheistic cultures, salvation is often seen as a thing that comes quickly, often
by having a transcendental experience and agreeing to some basic doctrines. In Asian
religions, with some notable exceptions, it is often believed that salvation will be a
long process: one's first attempts at personal and spiritual reform may in fact be
disasters. It is noted by many Gurus and Lamas and Masters that a new spiritual
practice, or an attempt to give up an addiction or to arrive at a place of sanity, may
be met with a series of near-fatal reversals. Salvation requires not only decades of
hard work but tons of luck and family support and community goodwill.

As long as people say 'I *should* have done it differently,' they are saying, 'I *could* have done it differently,' which translates to mean that they actually have power over their disease. *They are secretly in control!*

And so they don't need the First Step, because they are not powerless.

Sneaky, huh? Sometimes it takes a few crashes for us to learn. Nelson did. A banker in the UK with a handsome professorial beard and rapid-cycling Bipolar Disorder, he recounts:

> "Second time around, I knew what was happening and I knew I needed help to get through it. I also knew that, this time, I wouldn't get through it by myself because it's a painful process and I couldn't face doing that alone again. Oblivion would be preferable."

The trouble is, admitting our powerlessness makes us feel hopeless and worthless. As if we ARE our weaknesses and nothing else.

Popular slang tends to support this point of view, which is unfortunate. People refer to us carelessly as 'loony' or 'nuts' or 'crazy' or 'ga-ga.' The inference is that we are broken everywhere; that there are screws loose all over the place. Nothing we think or feel or do can be trusted for a minute. In fact, we really ought to just go jump in the trashcan.

But you are more than a walking-around broken brain. As you work the Steps and your spirit starts to stretch, you will feel this for yourself. In the meantime, there are things you need to know.

You are not a machine. There is more to you than the nuts and bolts of your central nervous system. There is nothing wrong with your knees or elbows. There is nothing wrong with your face, your IQ is intact (chances are it's higher than average), and so is your reproductive system. Even if you are seriously handicapped, there are still a lot more parts of you that *do* work than parts of you that *don't*. If that weren't true, you wouldn't be alive.

And your character. You have tons of character.

The fact that you're reading this, for instance, says that you are a diligent person with a serious interest in your own evolution. You are willing to look in your own dark closets. That's admirable, and that's just the start.

Most of the PASC I know are all of the following: brave, persistent, compassionate, resourceful, and humorous (how could we survive if we weren't humorous?). Many are startlingly original and creative. Most have depths and endurance that any guru would envy. Don't these sound like good qualities? The qualities of someone you'd like to know?

Well, now you do.

Give yourself credit. Right now, exactly the way you are, you're OK. In fact, you're admirable.

As Nelson puts it, "I am probably a stronger character because I know my limits, and understand why I change as I do, why I can be a Mouse or an Ox."

*   *   *   *

So. You're a terrific person but you're powerless. Nothing you do can change that or fix it or make it look better on your résumé.

Good. We're getting somewhere.

Now, about that word 'unmanageable,' as in "our lives had become unmanageable"...what does it mean? Of course, in Buddhism, the entire human condition is considered unmanageable. But in your personal life, how bad does it have to get before you confess, as the Step asks you to, "this is unmanageable"?

Think about Gordon. A young, raven-haired guy with the sort of face that attracts people naturally, and an intelligence that produced powerful, moving poetry. At first he only had a problem with Depression. Then it got worse, and the medicines didn't seem to help; so, he lost his first (and only) job and was forced to go on Welfare. While the government hemmed and hawed and refused to help pay for medicines, he started to hear voices. He thought the police were watching him and had put microphones in his house. He kept looking for them. The end diagnosis was Schizophrenia.

He couldn't work anymore, and he'd only just had his first job. That meant little money. He got eviction notices. He moved to a seedy residential hotel. His bathroom sink was *the* sink. His window looked out on an airshaft. He had one burner and cooking pot and lived off fast food. He was not a tough guy; and he became afraid to walk around in his questionable neighborhood. Later, the medicines blew him up from a sleek 140-pound fellow to over 300 pounds, none of it muscle. Though the medicines helped him a little with his symptoms, he couldn't find the combination of drugs that allowed him to function at anything like a normal social level. He was 23 years old.

This is unmanageable, don't you think?

Or Sandy, who didn't become ill until she was almost thirty. One day without warning, she started having Mania. By the time the episode was under control, she had lost her husband of many years and her excellent career.

Eventually she went back to school, got a degree in social work, and found a plum of a job in her new field. No sooner did she start work than she began to hear voices. Not just one, but a crowd-full. All day. Most of them were malignant. Many of them told her to kill herself. She left the job. And Social Security told her that she had been working too long: she was no longer eligible for benefits.

This is unmanageable, too.

These brave folks function against amazing obstacles. They are delightful company with fascinating interests and minds. And they don't stand a chance in the workaday world.

When you are living with special chemistry, you are dealing with something unpredictable. Any action you take, no matter how logical or well-planned, can be mercilessly undermined. Your alternate biology introduces a random element into every plan you make.

Vivien told me, "I have my birthday coming up in September. I'm seeing my daughter; we're going to a concert…and, um, I'm just praying that I'll be fine for that day." She adds, "People think, OK, you're taking your pills, you're doing this, you're doing that, you're FINE. But that's not always the case."

In other words, life with mental illness is inherently unmanageable.

We try to manage it anyway. That is human nature. It is not, however, the nature of the Twelve Steps. What you get depends on what you want. You can have reality, bad as it is, and the efficiency that comes with the truth. Or you can have wishful thinking, and the occasional, tight, tense feeling that THIS time you've got it right. Maybe. For a month or two. And then things will fall apart again. That is the nature of life when you are PASC.

Eddie Smith describes the futility of trying to 'control' such a life with this metaphor:

> "Most people that I see are complete and utter control freaks...me, I'm able to be a trooper under all possible conditions...some things I see in my life are meant to [be] lessons. And other things, the reason they don't look like lessons, after almost 50 years, is because they're not lessons...and if it's a lesson at all, it's an emergency evacuation order!

> "Like, there's a hurricane coming, and it's not a wonderful sign to me, it's a fucking hurricane. And its purpose is to come and fucking kill you. That's what they do, and that's what they're about. It's not a poem...There's a lot of people who literally – and this was true in Katrina, it was true in Andrew, it's true in every hurricane – *stand* there. National Guardsmen are trying to *drag* them out of the house, and they're holding them off at gunpoint, and finally the National Guard say, 'Okay.' People who die, every year, because literally a hurricane is coming and they will just stand there and say, 'God will reveal'...or whatever."

Some of us take a while to get the message that things are never going to be 'fixed.'

Let's pick on me for a while.

I've been addicted to drinking, sex and love, codependence, credit card debt, and several other things. With the Twelve Steps all those things gradually got better. But my PASC problem got a little more debilitating every year. First I had to quit working full-time. Then I lost my part-time job. Then the job after that. Soon I went bankrupt.

Broke, I moved to a neighborhood where drive-by shootings were normal. The apartment manager had a locked phone because he used to make molesting phone calls. I lost my boyfriend, because oddly enough he didn't like me yelling at him abusively whenever I had symptoms. Money got even worse, and I moved into somebody's back bedroom. From there I moved to a garage. But I couldn't stop being Bipolar and mean, and my last friends walked away.

Yet I was working on my Twelve-Step program all this time. So what am I saying? That the program failed me?

No. I'm saying I failed to apply the program where I needed it most. I never even thought to apply it to my special chemistry. Somehow, I figured that was a separate issue, one that did not interest God[3] and had nothing to do with recovery.

Well, why did I do that?

After all, hadn't the program quite literally saved my life? It had. Didn't the Twelfth Step clearly state that we are to 'practice these principles in *all areas* of our lives'? Yes, it did.

My problems were more personal: Embarrassment. Stubbornness. Plus a dose of good old-fashioned denial.

For one thing, I argued to myself, the Twelve-Step Fellowship was all about abstaining. Not drinking. Not debting. Not throwing myself into yet another compulsive relationship. Etc., etc., etc. I believe this is a very common view. Relief from addiction is enough to keep us satisfied. As a system of

---

[3] Or as a Taoist might say, was outside the Flow of the Universe. If the Universe is an Organism, part of our insanity might have to do with always feeling 'outside' and not within the Great Organism.

abstinence, however, the Steps did not seem like an appropriate approach to dealing with special chemistry.

Then there was the problem of Meeting etiquette. Some groups are very precise about what is and is not proper to share at group level; others are more liberal, so long as they are clearly Twelve-step issues. I didn't want to be 'rude.' I didn't want to take up people's time with something so 'irrelevant.'

One of the strongest psychological advantages of the Anonymous programs is that they allow everyone to belong somewhere. Whatever we've done, 'however low we have sunk,' as they say, someone is sure to have done the same thing. We 'hear our own story', we feel relieved and accepted, we are OK and human at last. No more shame and hiding. We are 'as sick as our secrets', right? That's what they say in the Twelve-Step Fellowship. You hear that all the time.

Well, I kept my secrets. And I was sick at heart.

What's clear to me now is that I was acting from misplaced pride. And the pride was driven by fear. *They'll know I'm not like anybody else. I will look ugly and strange and scary.* **They will not like me anymore**.

And if I can't belong *here*, for god's sake, where else can I go?

Nope. Telling the truth was just too dangerous.

So I went on my way, feeling just that little extra bit too weird, afraid to ask. I was resentful that I couldn't get my needs met. I became suspicious of all advice. They just didn't *know* what it was really like. They couldn't *understand* my special, unique, impossible problems. Their solutions just wouldn't work for me...which was a good excuse not to follow advice...and I found myself attending fewer and fewer meetings.

In short, I stopped thinking the rules applied to me.

Predictably, I ended up psychotic and in the hospital again, for the first time since my sobriety date (oddly enough, almost on the anniversary).

Even then, I didn't get it. I came out with a brand new set of medications, completely stabilized for the first time in my life, and I thought this was IT. I had finally gotten what I needed to be sane.

Within six weeks, I was right back to the chaos where I started. Medicines or no medicines, I could not maintain peace of mind without spiritual sanity. Well, I only knew about one reliable road to spiritual sanity. And I finally got humble enough to try it.

So it worked. Just the way it had always worked.

Why was I surprised?

We waste half the power of the Steps when we use them only as a band-aid. We waste most of the potential of our lives when we fight the unbeatable.

Try admitting you are up against the impossible, that you've been seeking to do something no human being can do alone.

When we take the First Step, we are doing something far more inclusive than admitting our powerlessness. We are welcoming ourselves back into the human race. It is freeing, it is relieving, it is something we have deserved for a long time now.

To be frank, this is also our duty to the human race. It's when people don't accept that they are PASC, think they can 'control' it all and refuse to take their medicines, that we end up with atrocities like the 32 people dead at Virginia Tech. This does not need to happen. We need to peel off our egos and do what needs to be done.

Outer Tips for Inner Peace

Strategy 1: Standard Medical Treatment

I'm going to point out some things that may seem obvious. But you'd be surprised how often folks who are obviously PASC just don't get the basics.

First of all, you must get medical care. This can be harder than it sounds. Finding care you can afford can be a problem. Getting people to help can be a problem.

Jessica, when she first tried to get help, was rudely shown the door.

> "I was up for review with SSI, I guess that was about 10 years ago....When I tried to go to the county [clinic], they wouldn't even see me and they wouldn't tell me why and they said they would throw me off the premises if I didn't leave.

> "I don't know why they did that. They wouldn't tell me why, why they wouldn't see me. They wouldn't tell me anything, so I got upset and angry, and they said they were gonna [throw me out].

> "It was really weird. It was like, 'Aren't you *used* to dealing with crazy people? Why can't you tell me what the hell is going on?' But they wouldn't."

When they did give her a list of Medicaid-approved doctors, she had trouble finding one who would see her:

> "So they gave me this list of Medicaid approved doctors. There were maybe four or five names on it and I called the one guy and he never called me back; I called the other and

he said, 'Well if you're just doing this because you're being reviewed for SSI then I don't think that this would work because we require a great deal of work ,' and I said 'I can do that' and he said, 'No, it just seems like you're trying to get over or something.'"

The third doctor she called remembered her from a previous SSI review and agreed to see her.

Typically we need a therapist for counseling and a psychiatrist for the medicinal side of things.

After you find your doctors, you have to make use of them!

Compliance

It is stupid not to take your medicine. Sorry to be so blunt.

There are lots of reasons people don't. I didn't, at first.

Firstly, we sometimes have this notion that if we're not taking any pills, we're not "really" sick. But that's ridiculous. If you refuse to take heart medication, but you keep having seizures, does that mean you don't "really" have a heart problem?

I understand why PASC people feel this way – I've been there – but it's a destructive fantasy. If you've read this far, you ought to know better.

What these people clearly don't know is how much better they can feel. I would rather have my fingernails pulled out than ever live in that hell before medicines again. Seriously.

Some PASC folks take their pills for a while, feel better, and then stop. Again, it's the hope that they "weren't really that sick" after all, or that it's over now and has gone away. Hello? You feel better *because* you took the medication, silly! It's not like an antibiotic, which you take till the bottle is empty and the infection is cleared. Your psychiatrist will be happy to slow or stop your pill intake if you really have gone into remission. It is very hard on your system to stop anything all at once if you're used to a regular dosage. Anybody who's ever decided to give up caffeine can tell you that!

Also, you're completely wasting your time if you go on and off when you "feel you need it." Again I'll use the heart condition as an example. Do you just take your medication when you "feel you might have a heart attack that day"? Hmmm?

Some PASC patients have the belief that the medicine doesn't change their behavior too much, and isn't worth the bother. They think they're perfectly OK without it.

This reminds me of a man I know who was diagnosed very late in life. He'd already shared many years of marriage with his patient wife. He started taking the pills under protest, decided that no one could tell the difference, and quit. He didn't tell anybody that he had quit. He figured no one would notice the difference, anyway.

Very soon his wife set him straight. "Either you go back on your medications or I'm leaving you!" she announced. She could tell he wasn't taking them, all right!

The sad truth is that we may *not* be the best judges of our own behavior. After all, you made sense to yourself all along, didn't you? If you've been PASC for a while, you may not be able to tell non-ordinary consciousness from ordinary consciousness. It's all normal and familiar to you. As long as your behavior makes perfect sense to you, you might not see the difference it makes in the outside world.

Those who have to live with you may be the only accurate barometer you have.

Hopefully this will not be true forever, but it often is in the beginning of treatment.

Here's the crux: as long as nobody thinks anything can be done, they have to take us or leave us. But once they know that we *could* be doing something to improve our behavior and we *won't* – hey, why should they stick around? If we're not going to even try, why should they waste their time and energy?

They might stick with us anyway. We could gamble on that. If they stand by us now, are we sure they'll do it forever? Tell me something: *Why should they?* It isn't fair. Not even to us, actually. They are just watching us let our life flow down the tubes.

Another objection special chemistry folk make to pills, especially with Mood Disorders, is that they won't be truly themselves anymore if 'their feelings are controlled by pills.' I have news: *your condition is not 'you'!* It is, in one way, like an overgrown vine on a tree. It has to be pushed aside if you want to see the trunk. You may value your altered states, and that's fine. But 'you' are more than any one state of consciousness. You need to be free to move between them all.

I'm personally delighted to find that the bitchy, promise-breaking, hostile behavior I displayed throughout my twenties was not 'the real me.' Thank God I had a chance to push it aside and find out who was under there!

The 'not-me' argument is similar to the fear of some artists that they will lose their creativity with their altered states. Some even think their special chemistry is the source of their creativity. Hogwash. We need *all* our states of consciousness to be good artists. We need the creator, yes – and we also need all the technical skills and mastery we've learned over the years to polish our work, as well as discipline to complete it. Those are very much rational-consciousness phases. A creative idea that is not executed, or is executed badly, is not what we are after.

We may feel a bit cut off for a while, it's true. But unless we are over sedated, the channels to our art will open again with exploration and nurturing. It's true there have been some very great 'tortured souls' in the history of art. And it's true that the viewpoint of an altered consciousness adds things to our perspective that cannot be gained any other way. The depth and scope of our work will be enhanced by our unique experiences. But we need not be forcibly sent there over and over again!

We need not be actively suicidal to write about Clinical Depression, for instance. The memory is enough. And if we are not being dragged into altered states randomly when we are trying to work, our productivity and quality are likely to improve. It is much better to have a choice about whether to trip off into another dimension, or stay at your desk or your easel and work.

You may feel that your chemical condition is actually a door to special spiritual abilities – say as a psychic or a channel or a shaman. I would certainly not dispute that with you. The world has had people like this for thousands of years. What I would urge is that you explore your possibilities under careful and close supervision. There is a time and a place for altered states. In the middle of a crowded intersection is not one of them. It is vital to our safety – and probably our income – to avoid random states that strike at inconvenient or dangerous times.

So I would still recommend a minimal course of medicine, and careful check-ins with a sympathetic doctor. Make sure you have plenty of support at hand as you explore. A nominal amount of medicine will probably not hinder you from going to other places in your mind. You will just need to learn the proper triggers, rituals, or ceremonies. Training in hypnotherapy, for instance, teaches one to enter a non-ordinary state that is therapeutic and useful. Aspiring shamans can also take classes. Other kinds of spiritual centers become available more and more in modern America.

I'd like to drop one word of advice that I hope will not offend these spiritual seekers. If we are known to have a mental condition, it's not wise to announce that we're "not really ill." People will misunderstand this as denial. Better, maybe, to say, "I've found some positive uses for my unique brain chemistry," or even, lightly, "Sometimes being crazy is an advantage." As PASC people, we have a very nervous audience. It's OK to be labeled eccentric. But we can't afford to lose our credibility. It's already fragile.

The Exceptions

There are exceptions to this, as there are to any rule.

When it comes to side effects, you have to make a judgment call. I strongly suggest you try other drugs recommended for your condition before giving up on your sanity! If every single anti-depressant destroys your sex life, for instance, that might be too high a price to pay. But usually, a switch to some other type of anti-depressant will fix the problem. (And, think about it: if you don't control your symptoms, are you going to have a sex life anyway?)

Another exception is if you feel you've been misdiagnosed.

No, I don't mean the knee-jerk reaction, "They're wrong! I'm not crazy!" *I am right and everyone else is wrong* is the default position for the human mind. That doesn't make it true.

But if you research the specific label they have given you, and it just doesn't seem to fit, I suggest getting a second opinion.

You can easily look up the various types of PASC in a book called the Diagnostic and Statistics Manual, or DSM. It will have a number after it, DSM IV or V for instance (as I write, we're coming up to the fifth revision). Look up the condition your doctor is assigning to you, and read the 'differential diagnosis' section. It will say something like, "Must have at least X number of the following symptoms," and then a list. If you can't find yourself on that list, it might be time for a referral.

Be aware that mistakes can happen if people are diagnosed *too quickly*. If you look over the DSM in detail, you will notice that a lot of those conditions can have multiple symptoms in common. It can be hard to distinguish one from the other, especially on short acquaintance, and mistakes do happen. My own therapist first decided I was Bipolar after a *year and a half* of regular weekly sessions. She got it right in one guess. But things can get messy if someone has only one or two meetings before diagnosing you.

On the other hand, just because they made a wrong diagnosis doesn't mean that you are 'well.' Chances are you do have a PASC problem if it's come as far as seeing the doctor about it. You still need medicine, the only important question is which kind.

If you read the entire DSM looking for what you do have, however, you will probably come away convinced you have every condition in the book. This happens to beginning psychology students a lot. It's because, as Dr. Kallinger said in his preface, we all have a little bit of every one of these behaviors in us.

One Special Exception

There is one other type of person I would exempt from my strict views about medication. That is the person whose health is so fragile that it starts to go seriously downhill when sufficient medication is taken.

I have met only one of these people in the last 20 years. He was born with one of the messier versions of cleft palate, the kind nurses and doctors refer to as a 'train wreck.' His condition involves eight separate birth defects, and that is not counting the various health problems that came along later. At one point, he found an eccentric and brilliant doctor who gave him some exotic mixture of medicines that made all his PASC symptoms go away.

The only problem was that within a few weeks he started losing his ability to talk or hear. And recently he found that another medication that helped made his blood pressure soar to truly frightening heights.

It's Eddie Smith. Did you guess?

Eddie still takes whatever miniscule dosages his body can handle. But lots of the time he just has to sit with his symptoms. I wouldn't want to live through his typical morning.

This is really not desirable, though some people seem to think that being pill-free is worth anything.

So if this is your level of physical fragility, you have my sincere sympathies, and I would consider you excused from taking your medications except on the most careful, delicate basis (e.g., at a fraction of the usual dosage, or only at particularly difficult times).

Otherwise, stick to the regimen. If your side effects are awful, talk with your doctor about substitutes; or you might want to look into alternative medicine as a supplement.

A Word About Mania

Mania is a special problem. People don't like to take medicine for it, because it feels so *good*! Mania gives you the great feelings that expensive recreational drugs only attempt to deliver. For as long as it lasts, you are happy and witty and brilliant and irresistible and invincible. You have more ideas than God, and you have enough energy to get it all done. Today.

Who wouldn't want that for free if they could get it?

A few years ago my psychiatrist remarked, "It's interesting. You're the only patient I know who doesn't like Mania." That's not exactly true. I love Mania. I'm not going to argue with you about how much fun it is. I've just learned to hate what it costs me.

I'm just going to be the wet blanket and ask: what about after?

Who is going to pay the hospital bill? The property damage? The $30,000.00 in credit card bills? The ticket back home from Russia, where yesterday it was such a good idea to go? How are you going to explain to your partner that it truly was only logical and fair that you sleep with their best friend? How are you going to explain to your next interviewer why you said what you said to your last boss in front of the entire staff?

How many times do you do this before you get tired of the cleanup?

I was Manic through most of my twenties, and it is amazing to me that I am not dead – probably murdered – while in the advanced throes of delirium tremens and HIV. I certainly would have earned it.

It's true that Manics are lots of fun at a party, and for a while people may tidy up the ruins for you. But what about when they quit, or die, or you get in too deep somewhere all alone with no friends and no working brain to help you get out?

Here's another question: Why would you want to be that much of a creep?

We didn't discover the right medical regimen for me until I was in my thirties. I have no friends left from my twenties. None.

No, wait. I have two. They both email, from many miles away, once or twice a year. I consider this very brave of them.

When it comes to Manic elation, less is definitely more.

Substance Use

I used to be a party girl. I'm not going to preach that all drugs and alcohol are bad. If a person with average brain chemistry needs a chemical escape once in a while, that's dandy. The only problem would be addiction, which of course is a major problem for anyone. That's a subject more than adequately dealt with by other authors.

But lots of PASC people like to keep their chemical amusements going even after they take meds. Sorry. That won't do.

I totally understand why they do it. I was actively alcoholic for a year even though I began taking pills. After all, drinking was almost the only time I felt good. As the old joke goes, "Why do you drink?" Answer: "I drink because I'm conscious."

It's called self-medicating, and it's extremely common. But it's a good way to go to hell by the short cut. Your pills won't work, plus you might die. That's about the worst side effect I can think of.

Here's the idea: our medicines are designed to nudge the very delicately balanced electrochemical reactions in our brains, and normalize them. If we use drugs or drink more than just occasionally, we are adding random chemicals to the soup. God knows what will happen next, but certainly *not* normalcy. Plus, we are making toxic waste dumps out of our bodies. How smart is that?

Look at it this way: We have trouble in the first place because our brains flip off into altered states unbidden. We shuffle to and from several different realities, which is why it is so hard to function in the world. If we use drugs or alcohol, we are adding *more* altered states, layer on layer. We are spinning further and further away from the world that most people live in most of the time.

How is that supposed to help things?

We need to *limit* or *manage* our altered states, not multiply them.

I'll be frank: I do sometimes allow myself a glass of champagne at weddings or New Year's Eve. But I did that only after more than 20 years of sobriety, and I thought about it very carefully first. I know the Alcoholics Anonymous crowd will consider me 'relapsed,' and they are entitled to say that. That is what they believe, and they have good reasons for believing it.

What AA does or does not think of me is not the point. My point is that five drinks a year – which is about what I take – are not causing a chemistry problem. Taking PASC meds doesn't mean we must never have a social glass of wine again.

It just means that as a PASC one needs to *avoid* recreational altered states. Our meds won't work, and we'll destroy our bodies (even if our relationships survive, which is something else again).

The only altered states I would heartily endorse are those caused by yoga, meditation, and other spiritual ventures. They are harder to come by, but they are the greatest highs and completely nontoxic.

Of course, if you are of the "Feel Good, Die Young!" school of thought, none of this applies.

But in that case, why are you reading this book, anyway? Hmmm?

STEP TWO

Find Your Spiritual Center

"Came to believe that a Power
greater than ourselves
could restore us to sanity."
- adapted from the Twelve Steps
of AA

STEP TWO

Even if you've been in the program for umpteen million years, you need to look at this step again. Behavioral illness – or PASC, if you will – puts a new spin on some of the basic issues raised by this Step.

For one thing, there's that demanding word 'sanity.' What do the writers mean by that? And do they know what the PASC person means by it?

For another thing, chances are you're a little angry with God. Why were you given this horrible problem, anyway? Why couldn't you have been born sane? Or, if you've been at this for a while, you may feel, "I've done it all, God. I've worked on my Twelve-Step program, taken my pills, gone to therapy, been in the locked ward – my part's done. Why don't you just FIX it?"

Vivien is quite frank about this anger.

> "Yeah, I do blame God. Though I love Him, I totally blame God for my illness. I believe if He wanted to, He could heal me right now. I've been suffering with this illness for 18 years. And it's hard. I'd like to not worry if my behavior is going to be strange."

When you really start looking at this Step from the vantage point of mental illness, you may find you need a thorough overhaul on what it really means.

Restored to Sanity

When I started working the Twelve Steps regarding mental illness, I ran into several immediate obstacles. One was that I couldn't actually be 'restored to sanity' – that is, I couldn't cease being Bipolar. What good (I reasoned) is all this work if it doesn't get me cured? I had to look at that for a while before I saw the hole in my logic.

The fact is, *nobody* gets *cured* by the Steps. The alcoholic is "recovering," but not "recovered." He or she is no longer getting drunk. The addict doesn't get non-addictive – s/he gets to stop taking drugs. And so on for the other Programs. We get happier, better, stronger, calmer...but we do not get to be a different person. We grow around our illness, grow above it, maybe even because of it. But it doesn't vanish.

So, okay. If I wasn't getting less than everyone else, then I didn't need to feel left out and resentful. I'd rather be well – who wouldn't? But being happier and stronger sounded like a good deal to me. It wasn't as if I had anything to lose by trying.

Yet the Step says clearly that we can be restored to sanity. What does that mean?

What is Sanity?

In the popular sense, 'sanity' is whatever the people around you think it is. It means conforming to the unwritten code of acceptable social behavior. In our culture, it is reasonable and rational for children (and some adults) to dress themselves as skeletons and witches and go out begging for candy on one particular night of the year. But just try that out within, say, a group of Aborigines. Some groups of people think it's rational to send thousands of men across half the world in expensive boats so that they can kill strangers. Some people think that drinking to oblivion is the only way to spend their Friday nights. Within their own contexts, these things are all perfectly logical and sane.

In this sense, "insanity" is any behavior that makes the folks around you confused, embarrassed, or uncomfortable.

Pablo is a gentle man in his sixties who has been plagued with Obsessive-Compulsive Disorder all his adult life. Here, he describes an experience he had in the '60s in the Midwest:

> "One of the most shocking cultural
> experiences I ever had was when I went back
> to Michigan in 1969 'cause my folks were going

to sell the family home, and there was stuff still in the [house]; and I had a pretty good size beard. And all of a sudden, I realized when I got off the plane that I was being stared at. Not only being stared at, there were people avoiding me. And I thought, 'What's wrong?'

"Suddenly I realized, 'It's the way I look'. I even went to our old neighborhood and knocked on the door of a neighbor, who was not my generation but he was a professor, and he opened the door, he looked at me and slammed the door in my face. And I thought, 'Wow! This is Midwest conservative America!' To them, I looked crazy."

But we need a more precise measurement than this to use in our daily lives.

The formal definition of sanity (according to the American Heritage Dictionary of the English Language, Houghton Mifflin, 1981) is:

SANE: (1) Mentally healthy; of sound mind. (2) Having or showing sound judgment; reasonable; rational [Latin *sanus*, sound, whole, healthy].

(Yes, I have more recent dictionaries, but I like this one. So there.)

Having covered the 'reasonable' aspect of this definition, what strikes me here is the use of the word 'whole.' A human being is not one-dimensional. Most thinkers have long divided us into three parts: body, mind, and spirit or soul[1]. At any given time, we are operating on any or all of these three levels. To be whole is to be integrated, to have the three working together in the appropriate proportions.

---

[1] that's if you concede the existence of a soul or Higher Power; we'll get to that. If you want to think about it right away, I'd highly recommend you look at Mel C. Thompson's addendum at the back of this book called Whose God?

Sanity can be divided up in much the same way. We can distinguish three levels of sanity: Behavioral, Psychological, and Spiritual. Let's look at each one in more detail.

(1) <u>Behavioral Sanity:</u> Or, if you prefer, functional or social sanity; the brain working normally. This is the one that medicine tries to reach. This is where the symptoms are. This is where people become afraid of you, or angry at you, or hurt. This is the level of day-to-day operation. Nothing at the present time can guarantee us this type of sanity; however the right combination of medicines sometimes results in prolonged periods of stabilization.

(2) <u>Psychological Sanity:</u> In our era, this has now become accessible to most of us. Psychological sanity, in its simplest terms, means the emotional and rational capacity to perceive and react to reality more or less as it is the majority of the time – i.e., without too much distortion.

It is worth noting that psychological sanity can exist even in the presence of mental illness. Your ego, superego, and id may be in perfect balance; your childhood and traumatic issues may all have been dealt with and brought into perspective; and yet your brain can refuse to function correctly. It is also worth noting, for those who haven't noticed, that there are large numbers of people in the world who are NOT psychologically sound, but are regarded as 'sane' simply by virtue of not possessing a known mental illness. The large number of rapists and perpetrators of incest, for instance, do not demonstrate any particular pathology.

Doesn't that make you think? What is the world calling 'sanity' if you can be 'sane' and still rape and murder?

Most of us, however, end up having problems in both the psychological and behavioral areas, for good reasons. Most of us have kinks and hang-ups which we came by honestly in the process of being knocked around by life. And if our brains keep giving us faulty information, we can be excused for an extra measure of confusion! That's where therapy comes in. It is not easy, but it is critical. We do not need old issues gumming up the works while we deal with neurobiologically faulty wiring.

So: we can have psychological sanity, with work.

The other thing which the Twelve Steps have to offer us is:

(3) <u>Spiritual Sanity</u> : This is what the Christian Bible refers to as 'The peace that passes all understanding'. It is the wordless, quiet space deep inside us that yoga, meditation, and numerous religious rituals are designed to help us reach. *This is the part of you that is not sick.*

Spiritual sanity is an 'It is well with my soul' frame of mind. It is the gut-level recognition that you are an integral part of the Universe; an abiding, inner balance. Sane actions proceed from this place.

Spiritual awakening (as promised in the Twelfth Step) is nothing more or less than becoming aware of this deep inner place, and nourishing it. This is not the property of any one religion.

When we first discover our inner soul, as addicts for instance, we usually find ourselves empty and screaming with need. Finding out how to heal that, and how to live from the quiet place, is what the rest of the program is about.

This is not easy. To be in balance even for a moment takes a certain internal stature. Those who reach this point on a regular basis possess spiritual greatness. (If you are in balance all the time, you have reached spiritual perfection, and you get to be Jesus or Buddha).

Most Westerners tend to be aware, to some degree, of their own individual importance, but fall wildly short in terms of recognizing their connections to the rest of the world and the universe. This is the famous 'self-will run riot' referred to in AA's standard text, fondly referred to as the 'Big Book.' It is an extremely common problem, and the one most often addressed by Western religion. That's why we hear so much about sacrifice and the Golden Rule.

In our century, however, attention is finally being paid to the other major imbalance: not loving ourselves enough or not valuing our part in the scheme of things. This is the great contribution of the 'Me Generation.'

Any given philosophy will tend to lean heavily to one side or another. But both points are of crucial importance. We are individually important, and we are also part of a whole.

The ability to *consciously choose* to work at these balances (or not) could be the famous 'knowledge of good and evil' that Genesis talks about, and the characteristic difference between humans and other forms of life.

Why Me?

There is another problem in surrendering to this Step, and it is a sticky one. If you have a chronic illness, and you have any gumption at all, you are probably pretty angry at God (or Allah, or Brahma, etc.) by now.

Vivien, a devout Catholic, spent a lot of time being angry at God, early on.

> "I used to be hard on God. When I was living with my parents, there was a cross from their bedroom. And I used to pick up the cross and say, 'I want you in Hell, the place you put me!' And then I threw the cross on the floor, and it broke. And then my mother said, 'Vivien, if you want to know a person who's been through Hell, just look at the person on the cross.'"

How could we NOT be angry at whatever or whoever did this to us? How could we trust It or even connect with It? Hasn't It messed us up enough?

There are two stages to internalizing this Step. One must believe (1) that there is some Greater Power with which one can connect; and (2) that it is essentially benign – i.e., that It has your best interests at heart. Very few people believe that they personally are the organizing principle of the cosmos. Most admit there is something greater and more powerful than they are, if it's only the mortgage company. But finding an acceptable rationale behind our sufferings is not easy. Philosophers have been playing with this question since the beginning of written history. Ultimately, the answer you choose will depend upon the type of Power you pick.

For instance, those who believe in reincarnation or Karma can reasonably conclude that they are working off post-dated debts from former lives (and thus have no need to complain), or working in this incarnation to learn a specific lesson.

Those who claim that we as humans are responsible for everything in our lives, right down to choosing our own parents, will recognize that they must have picked their particular handicaps for the lessons that they offer.

Nelson takes the entire 'why me' question impersonally:

> "I have mixed feelings about Divinity. If there IS a God, I suspect it is as the Hindus and Buddhists would have it, that everything is a manifestation of God. Hence, there is no 'personal' God that does things to people from on high. Indeed, what happens in the Universe CAN be explained as 'accidents' because the Universe is infinite; and with infinity, every improbability becomes a probability at some time, some where."

If you do favor a personal god, then clearly S/he had an objective in creating you this way, whether you understand it right now or not. This is an attractive position. It's usually not hard, if we take the long view, to find some way in which we have indirectly benefited from almost any kind of experience. Much of what we learn from our special chemistry brings us more than just pain: it brings a depth and scope of human experience not to be gained in any other fashion.

Vivien, for instance, says she learned to "…Listen. To the Inner Voice. Back then, I was hearing two voices…there was that voice that told me to go out and meet [her guitar teacher]… and starting right after that I'd hear a voice of reason. 'Vivien, no. He is just a human man. He doesn't know what is going on with you. Go ahead and do what you need to do. Take care of yourself.'" Unfortunately, she says, she learned to trust the second voice too late. By then, the teacher she was wandering all over the Mission to find had stopped talking to her, and she had been thrown out of the music studio.

But she has learned that lesson. Being able to hear your voice of inner sanity above all the other noise is no small gift. It is one some people never learn at all.

In my own case, I was born with precious little patience or compassion. I judged everybody, and I judged them harshly, from a hard, black/white place. (Once upon a time, in about my third year of therapy, I said, "Nancy, exactly what is it that we're doing here?" She said, "We are expanding your gray area.")

Whatever I know about kindness, I learned from my special chemistry. It forced my awareness of human weakness. It proved to me that sometimes people are powerless over what they do. I came to understand: I am certainly not the only one who's powerless to make her body conform to her heart's highest standards.

Lisa answered the 'Why me?' question this way:

"I believe in God unfailingly. I do not blame God for anything. Is there a good reason for my illness? Who can really know? Possibly, my soul agreed to accept this burden before my physical birth. Perhaps it's a trial to further my knowledge and enlightenment. Or maybe it's all random, and you have no choice but to take what you get—the possibilities are endless. I do believe that there is a purpose to everything, but I also believe that it's not our place to understand everything during our physical life."

And if you have faith in something less specific, such as Nature, the Universe, the Cosmic Will or what-have-you, you probably realize that you were simply in the wrong place at the wrong time. If you stand in front of a tidal wave, you get wet. Nothing personal.

The important thing to know is that, when you follow the Steps, you can be as mad at this Force as you want to – and it will still work for you.

Shanna, our teenage Bipolar interviewee, frankly admits that belief gives her some problems; in fact, it's historically a problem with other PASC members of her family.

"I don't know if it's because of the Bipolar Disorder, but to be completely honest, I have a harder time believing in God. But I do. I make myself, pretty much. I do believe in God, as far as God goes, but some of the – my grandma is Schizophrenic and she has some really hard times with God, because every time she goes to church, she has mental breakdowns and tries to kill herself and stuff.

"Momma pretty much went through a spell where she was afraid we'd end up like grandma. She didn't really want – like, she wanted us in church, but she was scared, I guess. So we didn't go to church for a while, but Momma would teach us. What we needed to know, she let us know.

"As far as God goes, I try. I know this is terrible, but my brother and my sister are like, 'why don't you ever do this?' or 'why don't you ever do that?' I had my reasons. But I don't know if this has anything to do with being Bipolar or not, but I hate praying in groups. I hate praying out loud. I just hate it. I mean, I cannot stand it. I just want to be alone, if I pray I want to be alone."

She has also spent time angry with God:

"When I was having breakdowns and stuff, I'd go to my room and I'd be, like – when I was having really bad things like [imagining] my dad dying, I would go to my room and say, like, 'If you take my dad, I'll never pray to you!'

> "I threatened God. I know that's not good and all, but I couldn't help it at the time."

Those with special chemistry particularly need a concept of the divine that is benign.

> "My mental stability, I don't know if it's like this now, but I used to could not handle – I think it's Hellfire and Brimstone? People talking about the end of the world scares the crap out of me. I can't handle it.

> "Like people talking about the world ending in 2012, I don't believe it. But when people do talk about it, I just start shaking."

So we can be angry, and we can be scared, and if we feel God is responsible, it's natural we're going to blame God and ask "Why?"

It has been said that recovery is a matter of continually trading in one set of problems for a *better* set of problems. I am suggesting that 'Who did this to me?' and 'Why me?' are not useful questions.

Pablo went through these questions, too.

> "You want to know what's wrong! I mean, that's a normal [feeling]– what I kept feeling – during all those years, I kept thinking it was only me. There was no one else in the world like I was. There was only me. And I was this weirdo, you know, that had this kind of problem – and why me? When you realize that it's a condition that other people have, too, it makes you feel better, in the sense that you're not alone; that it's not that abnormal; in the sense that there're thousands of

other people with exactly the same problem. Once I began reading...it didn't seem like such a hopeless, horrible thing that had somehow been put upon me. Or that you were being *punished* or something.

"...But also, when I began to realize that this is most likely inherited through the genes, and that the Obsessive-Compulsive [Disorder] is much more in tune with the primitive brain – this is the way the primitive brain functions, as opposed to the modern intellect brain – I did go through a period where I felt like I was being punished. Something was punishing me for this. But not God. I did not go and say, 'it's your fault or your fault or your fault'. I [do] have the tendency, even today in talking to Mom, to say, 'Well, it came through the genes.' In that way you can say, there's the fault, but it's not part of the blame. You know, [Mom's] not to blame for it, nobody is. It's so easy to want to blame. Because it does make you feel better in a way, in the short term.

"The thing that helped [me] try to concentrate more on the *positive* side was that if the primitive brain was much more in charge, and I could learn to control that, then I could tap into the *good* part of that."

The thing that makes a difference is asking, 'What do I do about it?' And this guides us straight back to the wisdom of the Steps. First we admit we can't do it alone. Then we start looking for someone else who *can* help. For many of us, that is a divine source, what the Steps refer to as 'a Higher Power.'

If You Don't Believe

The majority of my interviewees did not believe in any particular religious system. Nelson had an interesting backdoor into Atheism:

"The Universe is infinite and, within infinity, every improbability becomes probable at some time, some where. So, do I feel there is a good reason for my illness? No! That's just the way the Cosmic dice fell."

Eddie doesn't really buy anybody's theory:

"The funny thing about the problem of evil is that the gurus and the Buddhists that all go through that somehow kind of say...that you sinned, or that [it's] your karma brought on by what you did, [accepting] the idea that there is a lesson.

"So: Okay. They started beating me with a stick, thirty years ago, chained me to a wall. Thirty years later, every morning, while I'm chained to the wall, they beat me with a stick. That's their plan forever.

"Well: it's totally reasonable? Probably not [laughter].

"So, being a trained philosopher, I can't really buy that. I'm just unable to. Not 'unable to' like I'm not strong enough to believe it. But the greater lesson theory – there's just too many instances where you have to try to suspiciously hard to *work* [at believing] it."

What may surprise you is that Eddie is nevertheless the most relentlessly spiritual man I know. He practices yoga and meditation, goes to a regular Zen group, and has written a number of hymns that have now been included in the Jodo Shenshu Buddhist canon. He does not buy anybody's theory in particular, but he finds enormous help in spiritual practices and rituals.

We are looking for results here, not adherence to any system.

If you can't or won't believe in any given system, but you still want the program to work for you, I suggest you take a look at the work of Carl Jung.

It was Jung who first suggested to one of the earliest Alcoholics Anonymous members that the key to lasting sobriety was "a firsthand religious experience." Why?

Jung believed, along with Freud, (and it is now overwhelmingly accepted in certain psychological circles) that consciousness existed on three different levels in human beings: the Waking Conscious, the Individual Unconscious, and the Collective Unconscious. This last contained prototypes for mythological and religious characters that have been embedded in humanity's psyche since ancient times. We all share them. And we use this material to construct our beliefs, our dreams, our characters. We are frightened by the same dark figures and forces. We are lifted by the same heroic visions.

Given this information, is it so surprising that many of the world's religions resemble each other in crucial ways? Is it any surprise that every race HAS a religion, whether all individuals adhere to it or not?

The point to note here has nothing to do with the correctness (or not) of any religion, living or dead. The point is that *the human brain is hardwired to work at its best when you believe in something larger than yourself!*

The fact is, this trend is so ingrained that you probably already believe in something or other, anyway. There is already some thing, idea, person or concept by which you measure yourself – an organizing principle around which you build your life, a standard by which you judge the worth of your existence. It might be Justice or Art or Activism. It might be

Financial Security, or the Sanctity of Family. It could be a woman or man, or the need for one. Reason and Science are very common Higher Powers. To some extent they have replaced religion in the modern world. Perhaps it is the political arena, or A Just Society. You may, in your condition, worship health or an elusive thing called 'Normalcy' or 'Happiness.' Certainly, if you have a dual diagnosis, you at one time placed alcohol or drugs in the 'God' position.

The important thing to get from this discussion is that 'the God space' never remains empty for long. It will always be filled by *something*, because that is the way we are constructed.

Never mind whether you call it God or Allah or the Existential Dilemma. If you don't know what you're living by, isn't it time you tried to find out? Isn't that what a genuinely logical, open-minded person would do?

After all, if you don't like what you see, you can always replace it with something better.

There is so much to this subject that I have not sufficiently studied, I admit. That is why I turned to the philosopher Mel C. Thompson to write <u>Whose God</u>? and I suggest you give this a good look. If nothing else, it is instructive to get an idea of the many things that people all over the world have chosen to believe with all their hearts. You need not choose any of them, but you can be clear about your own position.

* * *

It is really not 'evil' or 'wrong' to go shopping for a Higher Power that you can believe in. Even the Christian bible says very clearly, "Work out your own salvation with fear and trembling." What is important is that you tap into something that is meaningful to you.

I am neither for nor against any established religion[2]. I do hope that my readers will forgive me for sticking to shorthand

---

[2] Including the dead ones of ancient Greece. It's recorded in the New Testament that one city had an altar inscribed "To The Unknown God" – just in case, in their endless pantheon, they had missed somebody! They might have it right, at that. Isn't God, after all, the Ultimate Unknown? Many religious groups today would benefit by adopting this sort of humility.

terms such as the Christian word 'God' once in a while. Christianity is, after all, the dominant belief in our culture; and I admit it is what I grew up with, so it is most comfortable for me. But please understand that I feel we are all included here, never mind how we approach the invisible or what language we may choose.

Those who find strength and surety in their church or temple should stay there, even though they may occasionally feel out of step with the rest of the world. The kind of inner stability we are after transcends all belief systems. We need not even believe in a 'self' or a 'soul.' Call it the Core, if you like. We need not know exactly what it is.

Nor am I saying 'pick what you like – anything goes!' The spiritual underpinnings of any life are a serious and private business. They call for the most rigorous honesty we can summon. Only you know where you are weak or nasty; only you know what touches you deep in your gut and inspires you to bring out the best you have.

The program does not insist that we choose any SPECIFIC path through the universe.

But it does insist that we CHOOSE.

We are going to be relying on that Power to help us discover everything that we are and become everything we can. To adopt somebody else's god, just to have one, is not only moral laziness; it will ensure that we never get what we need. Not from Twelve Steps or from 12,000.

As special chemistry folk, we sometimes have to tolerate a lot of dependency – on our pills, on our doctors, on the government and the welfare system, on the continued help and understanding of those around us. We may even have to take their word, sometimes, about reality itself.

But letting someone else choose our Higher Power is not a luxury we can afford.

Free Choice

There may not be any religion that completely satisfies you. That is OK, too. If America's Founding Fathers had been a little more careful, they might have said, "Freedom of Spiritual Beliefs" instead of "Freedom of Religion." Many people are finding in our age that no existing system quite fits. They pick a fact from here, a ritual from there, an idea from a far-flung culture. Or they may make up their own wild and crazy system that no one on earth shares.

There is one thing I believe with all my heart. That is that in this human body, with only five or six senses, we are not equipped to absolutely know The Truth about the universe. Even scientists admit that they can neither prove nor disprove the existence of God (or whatever you wish to call It).

So the concept I'd like to agitate for is tolerance of other beliefs. For one thing, it is the American way, and the way of the Twelve Steps. For another, any other policy leads to war, torture, hatred, the Spanish Inquisition, witch trials, and – most lately – terrorism.

It is perfectly acceptable to share your beliefs – if you wish – under appropriate conversational circumstances. It is another thing to harangue and harass people and try to write your own beliefs into law.

If your church has a missionary tradition, that may be difficult to accept. But I would point out that Jesus himself did not go door to door trying to convince people that only he could save them. He offered what he had, and crowds came to *him*, even out in the wilderness.

Believe what you want. Let others do the same. That is what loving adults do. And it is, by our Constitution, the 'American Way.'

Outer Tips for Inner Peace

Strategy 2: The Smart Patient

Jessica, the graduate student from the last chapter, is unhappy with her doctor and feels trapped.

"I don't like the medicine he prescribes for me. He frustrates me because he prescribes too many and he doesn't change when he's supposed to. I'm kind of scared of him and afraid he'll get me kicked off SSI if I stop seeing him. So I keep seeing him. Also he gives me Ativan which helps me with my Anxiety attacks and I'm afraid another doctor won't give me those. He's had me on the same thing for, like, 10 years now. You know the doctor, like, he talks to me *down*, it just seems...So I keep doing this. But I have my doubts about him."

The sad truth is that if you are on Medicare or Medicaid, you may not have a wide choice of professionals. These programs do not pay well currently and involve cumbersome paperwork, so many doctors will no longer deal with them at this writing. It is important to choose a doctor you feel comfortable with, though, if you have a choice. Sometimes even in a clinic that is highly limited or overburdened, it is possible to simply switch to another doctor. This will often solve the problem. I have had good doctors and bad, and I can tell you it is worth the extra effort in terms of health and peace of mind to find one you can work with. I now take an hour's train trip and a half hour walk to see my psychiatrist, because he is the best one I have ever dealt with, and the one I trust. So what if I can't afford him and it's a hassle? This is my sanity we're talking about, my daily ability to function and have friends.

Once you have a psychiatrist and a therapist – whether by Medicaid, sliding scale (worth checking into, if your cash is limited: many doctors will do this), or private practice – you must learn how to work with them.

You must be honest with your medical provider. You should be doing that anyway as a Twelve-Stepper. The Steps call for a lifestyle of 'rigorous honesty,' familiar words to those of us who have been in the program before.

I know that sometimes we're not in good shape to communicate. Make a list in that case, or bring along a friend or spouse who knows what's been happening, and what you want said.

It is crucial to participate in your own healthcare. I can't say that often enough. If your prescriptions don't seem to be working properly, tell your doctor. S/he may recommend that you try them for a while longer. This doesn't always mean you're being given the runaround, or that they don't care. Some medicines take weeks or even months to build up to a functional level in your blood stream or other tissues. Sometimes a dosage change of even half a milligram can make all the difference. On the other hand, if you keep having to change from one drug to another, try to be patient. It can sometimes take years to find the perfect combination or dosage for your particular body and mind. In my case, it took eight. In Vivien's case, 18 years have failed to turn up a dosage or combination that will make her function at the level she remembers. Improvement and response are highly individual, and frankly, science hasn't been working on this for very long.

In the end, you may just have to settle for some side effects that are less than comfortable. It's a judgment call. How much are you willing to put up with to be sane? What's it worth to you to think calmly and peaceably and be able to live the rest of your life outside a hospital? It could be worth considerable sacrifice.

You are not a passive pill-taking zombie, however. If something persists in not working or gives you side effects you *can't* live with, speak up! If the doctors don't seem to be listening, tell them again! If you've really given it your best shot, if the doctor doesn't seem to know you're alive, go find another one. One who will treat you with the intelligence and respect that you deserve. You are not an idiot, no matter what might be wrong in your brain. You and you alone have the inside scoop on how well the treatment is working.

Lisa gives this counsel:

> "My advice to the mentally ill population is to insist on an accurate diagnosis. If what is being done doesn't feel right, it probably isn't. It's okay to want to feel better, there's nothing at all selfish about that. You may have forgotten what it feels like to feel normal, or you may never have known, but your intuition knows."

And don't hesitate to ask questions. If you want to know more about a medicine, ask your physician to show you the Physician's Desk Reference, which describes meds and their effects in detail (perhaps more detail than you'll want!). Or you can go to the local library and look it up. It's a good idea, anyway, to read up all you can on your own disease. Educated questions get better responses.

Use the input of people around you. They can tell when you're getting off base, even though you may not be able to. If a lot of friends seem to be reacting strangely or 'unfairly,' it may be that you are having trouble seeing reality straight up. Just yesterday I found that I had been haranguing a bank for a mistake when in fact I was the one who was confused and wrong. After decades of the right treatment, that still happens once in a while.

Check with the people closest to you, privately – the people you trust. Find a code phrase, if necessary. I usually suggest that my partner warn me that I'm 'not acting quite like myself today' – a nice, inoffensive phrase – and ask me if I am OK. Then, it is up to me to decide what's required. Maybe I need to take an anti-psychotic. Maybe I just need to go somewhere quiet and rest for a while. Or maybe I'm upset for a perfectly acceptable reason, and there's nothing wrong with me at all. That happens, too.

What if you don't trust anyone around you? Sometimes we are trapped in situations where those closest to us are not entirely sane themselves, or are manipulative or selfish, and don't really have our best interests at heart. Maybe they can't, because what we do affects them too closely. It's a sad truth that some of us are mangled because we came from pretty mangled households in the first place. And if we can't earn our own living, perhaps we cannot leave.

That's why you need a therapist. The heart of therapy is *to have a healthy relationship.* To have someone in your life who will always listen, accept unconditionally whatever you do or say or feel, and whose only interest is for *you* to be happy and healthy. If you have that model in your life, even once, you can learn to build other relationships like it, and to make better choices about whom to have around you.

Once you have a grip on what reality is *supposed* to feel like, you will have a clue to when you are *not* operating within healthy limits.

But you do need at least one person to model complete acceptance of you. You will start to respect yourself, and have a feel for when you are truly being yourself, and when you are a little bit off track. That is the core reason I recommend therapy so highly, regardless of what you do or do not find out about your childhood and other issues.

The point is, people around you can give you useful clues; and with this help, prevention can be learned. More about prevention in Step 10.

Other Medical Issues

Beware that you do not blame everything that goes badly in your body on mental illness. Other things can go wrong. The mistake is to think that all uncomfortable symptoms come from either your disorder or your psychiatric medicines.

I have done this twice, which is why I warn you. In my thirties my libido suddenly and inexplicably disappeared, and I blamed my medicines. I had my psychiatrist change a number of prescriptions, and he even apologized to me, thinking his prescriptions had caused the problem. But it turned out that the real reason was my new birth control shots, and no one had warned me about this possible side effect. Even after I quit the injection, my sex drive did not come back for a whole year. By then of course, the relationship I had been trying to nurture was over.

More seriously, I have suffered constantly from fatigue and low energy for the last 12 years. In the end I was sleeping as much as 16 hours per day; sometimes even a night, the next day, and then the following night. Yet I was still exhausted. This pattern of behavior eventually made employment (and many other things) impossible.

I was told this was 'Residual Depression.' The various doctors I saw had nothing else to suggest once we had checked my thyroid and iron levels.

One day in 2008, my husband asked me, "Did you know that you sometimes stop breathing when you sleep?" It turned out I had severe sleep apnea. My body was partially waking me up 40 times *an hour*, because I could not breathe properly. No wonder I was tired! But if my husband had not tipped me off, my physicians would have gone on assuming they already *knew* what was wrong: I was Bipolar, so fatigue had to be from Depression.

Don't be paranoid about your body, but be aware that it is complex; you may have to look at other causes than the 'obvious' ones.

If You Run Out of Medicine

Some pharmacies may give you a day or two's supply of an emergency medication if you can't get through to your doctor (show them, with the empty bottle, that you *do* have a prescription). This works best if you regularly go to one pharmacy and they know you there.

I advise you to make sure your pharmacy is on a nation-wide computer system. If you are traveling, and you run out, you will still be able to get your medicine because the local pharmacy has the same records as your hometown.

One Last Tip

Never *ever* go anywhere without a supply of pills. I don't mean you must cart dozens of prescription bottles around jangling in your purse or briefcase. I mean, count out the pills you will need each day and put them in a little tiny container and stick it in your pocket or purse. I strongly recommend having an *extra day's supply* with you *at all times*.

Life is surprising. You do not know when you are going to be unexpectedly stuck somewhere for a while, even overnight, by injury or accident or a car breakdown or your ride flaking out. If you are prone to Panic Attacks or psychosis, you don't know when things could suddenly turn very weird. You *must* be prepared. The chances of someone being nearby who can actually help you are very slim.

I started this practice in 1989, when a local freeway collapsed in an earthquake and people were pinned under the structure for over 24 hours. I thought, 'What if that had happened to me and I had no medicine?' A trauma like that would have driven me straight into psychosis (otherwise known as hell). So I started carrying a pill box that fit into a pocket of my wallet. I have never been sorry.

If the injury or accident scenario doesn't convince you, think of this common situation: your pills have run out. You don't have a refill. No one can reach your doctor. Wouldn't it be helpful to have an emergency supply? Or what if you simply forget your normal pills and you are stuck somewhere away from home and starting to lose your sense of reality? If your emergency pill box is in a pocket, you are still safe.

Would you rather carry a pill box, or explain things to the police?

STEP THREE

Commit to Living From That Center

"Made a decision to turn our will and our lives
over to the care of this Power
as we understood It."
adapted from the Twelve Steps of AA

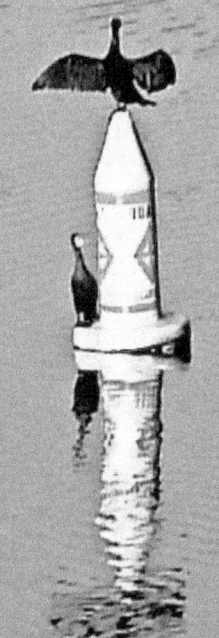

STEP THREE

This is my favorite step, because this is where things start happening. This is where one actually starts to see results and feel better.

It's also the one I have to do most often, because I'm not very good at it. Letting go of the reins comes pretty unnaturally to most of us.

But this step has also been widely misinterpreted by a lot of very sincere individuals. *It is not a call for unconditional surrender to forces unknown.*

Does this surprise you?

Look at Step Three carefully. It does NOT say you should turn your will and life over to a Higher Power. It says to *the care of* a Higher Power. This is not semantic hair-splitting. It's a very important difference.

In the first place, what is our 'will'? Isn't that a bad thing? Doesn't the Big Book of Alcoholics Anonymous say that we get into messes in the first place by having too much of it?

Well, yes – and no. What the text actually says is "self-will *run riot.*" In other words, pursued to a blind and obsessive degree: beyond all logic or practicality; without reference to the real world and the compromises that world calls for.

I'm reminded of a scene from an old TV show, "Hogan's Heroes." A group of Allied prisoners of war are putting together an airplane in the secret tunnels under their barracks. One of them calls, "Colonel, what do I do now? This piece just doesn't fit!" Hogan takes a quick look, picks up a sledgehammer, and rams the peg into place by sheer force. "Now it fits," he says.

THAT'S self-will run riot. Never mind if the plane will fly. At least he got his way!

But having a will – a normal-sized one – is a simple and necessary thing. It is, in fact, a non-negotiable part of the human package. No matter how much you 'turn it over to God,' as Twelve-Step members are always advising, there are still going to be things we are willing to have happen, and things we aren't.

This is not necessarily a bad thing.

Browsing through several dictionaries, I find that a 'will' is a determination, a choice, a desire or wish, a set purpose. There is nothing wrong with any of those things. It's hard to see how anyone could get across the street without a choice or a set purpose. All the details of our lives at any one time are the sum total result of the conglomerate things we are willing to do, and the actions we're taking to get there.

If a person gives up her will and her life, what has she got left? Of what use would such a creature be, to God or anyone else, having no desires but a request for the Universe to please take over and do everything? That is neither good ethics nor 'good program' (a Twelve-Step fellowship phrase for doing a good job working at your steps). No: that is parasitism. It turns humankind into a large, whiney child, and God into a cosmic vending machine!

Even the open-ended 'Power of your choice' recommended by the Twelve Steps can be misinterpreted in this regard. Jessica explains how her prayer life is constrained by popular program notions:

> "I believe I can ask God for things, to help me with things. Sometimes I'm not sure if He's listening. I sometimes feel that's my fault because I don't pray enough for other people. I pray too much for myself.
>
> "I think I got that from AA. They say you're not supposed to be self-centered and so I figure I should pray for other people instead of myself because otherwise it's self-centered...

I have trouble choosing how I'm going to pray...It's just hard. I don't know how well it works for me having a God that's dictated by AA, either.

"I keep having guilt feelings because I'm not praying enough for other people. Then it's just one more thing to be Anxious about."

A Higher Power dictated by some source outside us is often a bad idea, even if that source is usually reliable. Our Higher Power must be keyed to us personally, and how we work. It must include *us* as part of the equation. If your concept of God does not resonate down to your bones, then you won't be able to follow it or count on it when the chips are down.

It is, in any case, impossible for a human not to have a will of their own. To pretend we don't, and to suppress our true wishes, leads not to peace but to the ugliest kind of spiritual underhandedness. If we want to live a life of rigorous honesty, as the Big Book recommends, we must start by admitting that we *do* want certain things. (Insisting that we get them is something else again.)

We can't fool our Higher Power about this anyway, so why try?

What the Third Step asks us to do is to decide, thoughtfully and consciously, that we'll turn our will (whatever it may be at that moment) over to the *care* and *review* and *approval* of our Higher Power. We ask, on an ongoing basis, to have our lives incorporated into the greater scheme of things. And it logically follows that we are asking to be shown a different way *if our wishes do not fit the Higher Power's plan.*

We are agreeing, in short, to follow directions if ours aren't right. That's hard for normal human beings, which is why we have to practice this Step over and over.

So how do we ask for direction, and how do we get the answers?

We pray.

How to Pray

Any old way you want.

Is that too simple an answer?

In the West, prayer generally has an active connotation. We put out a request into the universe. In Zen Buddhist meditation, no requests are generally put out to any being, or even to the cosmos in general. However, there is a practice of deep listening. And this could be a type of prayer, simply listening to the universe; not necessarily putting forth one's own thought or opinion, but just awaiting what comes in a very alert manner. Westerners might perhaps call this 'listening prayer.'

At its base, prayer is nothing more than communication with the Higher Power of your understanding. That means any way that works for you is valid. But that's not what many of us were taught.

The God of my childhood (and perhaps of yours) had very definite ideas about how He should be approached. There was usually a paragraph of flattery before one could get down to business, and more at the end; at which time, one used the code word 'amen.' This struck me at the time as petty, or even vain. It was years before I understood the purpose of this manner of address.

The program, too, contains a number of suggested prayers, including the Lord's Prayer, borrowed wholesale from what Christians call the New Testament. The Serenity Prayer and the Third-Step Prayer (as derived from the AA Big Book) are two others that spring to mind.

But the program departs radically from religion in two important ways:

1) You decide what your Higher Power is

2) You communicate to it as seems best to you

I have prayed silently while standing on crowded busses. In tears on my apartment floor. Yelling and shaking my fist at the ceiling of the apartment. I have tried any number of approaches, from pleading with promises of good behavior, to telling God just where He got off and what She could go and do with Herself. The interesting thing is, no matter to whom or how one prays, one gets results.

A sincere desire to contact a Higher Power seems to be all that is required of us. Mark Twain once defined prayer, via <u>Tom Sawyer</u>, this way:

> "Tom's heart ached to be free, or else to have something of interest to do to pass the dreary time. His hand wandered into his pocket and his face lit up with a glow of gratitude that was prayer, though he did not know it."
>
> - Mark Twain, <u>Tom Sawyer</u>, Chapter 7

The Christian Bible also says something similar, claiming that "We do not know how to pray worthily...but his Spirit within us is actually praying for us in those agonizing longings which never find words." (Romans 8:26 and on, Phillips Version).

There is something to be said for traditional prayer. When we decide to accept a Higher Power's guidance, we are moving into a realm of great uncertainty. We are giving up the right to insist on our plans. We are accepting a new way of life that demands that we NOT always know what happens next; we are admitting that we don't even know what would be <u>best</u> to happen next.

Traditional religion would call this faith or humility. We don't have to call it that, if we'd rather not. Alcoholics Anonymous literature refers to open-mindedness and willingness, or 'teachability.' These words are equally good descriptions of what the Third Step is aiming for.

Anyone who's seen much of life will tell you that the idea that we control our lives is an illusion. There IS no security, safety, or even much self-determination.

Eddie illustrates our lack of security:

> "...this happens all the time in the world. There are perfectly healthy people whose skills have been tapped out – everybody

has a different level of total body capacity, total mind capacity – and there are people who have literally thought of every angle they can think of, and done everything that they can physically do, and the answer is: 'That's cool that you did all that. It won't be enough for survival in this situation, sadly. But: solid effort!'

"There are parts of Afghanistan where, right now, next to the old Buddhas that the Taliban blew up, well, there were a bunch of Muslim people who were living off those Buddhas. Tourists would come and see them; they had little tourist-y businesses. So when the Taliban blew up the Buddhas, all these people had no conceivable way of earning a living. There's no economy in Afghanistan unless you're, like, a heroin grower – or if you have, say, an exotic rug manufacturing plant, with ancient craftswomen hand-sewing...you know. Other than that, there's kind of no plan, in Afghanistan.

"So, they had these tourist deals. That got fucked up. So these people are living in caves, and there's literally nothing. There's no economy, and there's no infrastructure, and no electricity and no plumbing of any kind. And there's no water. You have to walk several miles to the nearest water each day, and back, just to not die of thirst. And in those caves, in the winter – 'cause it's like a zillion degrees below zero in the winter – they have to gather firewood *if* it's not completely picked dry that week. If it is, maybe they'll die of heat, or die of exposure, or die of thirst, or die of hunger, or just work so hard for one cent an hour until they drop dead.

"So the greatest effort on earth is often not sufficient socio-economically, even though your mother loved you, and your dad raised you honorably, and you had loving support the whole time and never had a psychiatric disorder. That in itself – and you're spiritually positive and everything – that does not guarantee your survival. The world doesn't know that. The world doesn't know that, all over the world, you could be completely psychically healthy, completely physically healthy, and spiral down to death because literally your best isn't good enough. Under the circumstances.

"Right, so even *if* you cured me of one physical or mental ailment or the other, the complex of my body and mind is such a train wreck that I'm at maximum capacity, and over-capacity, most of the time. I'm at the verge of going nuts. I say over-capacity because capacity is *sustainable*.

"Say an elevator can carry 11 people? Well, it really could carry 20 people for one day, but then the cable's going to start fraying.

"So what they mean is, if you keep it down to 11 people, you could do this for a year before you have to replace the cable.

"So [for the mentally ill] it's all just completely unsustainable."

Sometimes our best effort is not sufficient to control our circumstances. Nobody is going to keep things under control if they are run over by a war, a tsunami, and financial collapse all at the same time. And no one is really in a position to guarantee that these things will not happen. Some people just have better odds, and they like to think they are 'safe.' Mental illness, in common with most other chronic and incurable illness, strips away that feeling of safety.

Most of the time, though, security is an illusion, plain and simple.

The problem is, most human beings cannot maintain a flexible attitude about their real level of control for more than a few minutes at a time.

This is where the old models of prayer come in: bowing to Mecca, kneeling in prayer, etc. They are designed to remind us how little control we really have, how desperately we need to trust a Greater Power to be healed. All those fancy words I disliked as a child are NOT to fill any need of God's for flattery or worship. They are for ME. They remind me, when I'm inclined to forget and try to give God directions, instead of asking for directions.

Set prayers are fine if they help us. Kneeling is great if it reassures you. Our Higher Power listens to whatever we say, however we say it, and works in our lives. It is our job, when praying, simply to open a channel so a Power can come in.

So do it however it makes sense to you. But do it.

What Happens Next

My father loves to quote Bible verses. One of his favorites is, "Draw nigh unto God and he will draw nigh unto you." That's basically it.

For some reason, the universe requires that we make the first move. But when we do, we wake up Something of great generosity and sometimes startling intimacy.

I originally started this paragraph with the phrase 'prayer works.' But that gives the impression that every time you pray you get what you want, which is demonstrably not true. So let me put it another way. Prayer always has some effect. You might say prayer influences things. It may not be enough to get the result you want. But it does have an effect on reality.

Why can I say this? Because it is beginning to be a matter of scientific evidence. Decades ago I read in *Psychology Today* about a very credible study which showed that patients who were prayed for by a group recovered an average of 15% more quickly than patients who were not: and this was true *even if the patient did not know about the prayers.* I have seen other quite credible studies of the kind over the years, and it fits in with my own observations.

Why would this be? Well, the best theory I can give you is that, as we are beginning to see from physics, thoughts are energy. And the universe is entirely made up of different forms of energy, whether conglomerated as matter or floating around free. So if we lather up enough energy, whether by intense prayer, or repeated prayer, or group prayer, we are causing eddies in the universe, so to speak. Kind of a chaos theory – the butterfly flits its wings in Madagascar and by a chain of events that can be infinitely long, a tidal wave is caused far away. That's my personal explanation. You're welcome to take or leave it.

For whatever reason, as millions of people can tell you, prayer does provoke an answer. The trick is in learning to listen for these answers. It is not helpful to expect literal hands stretching down to solve our problems. The universe is more subtle than that.

Lisa wrote me a third-person story about her prayers as a child:

"In the magic of childhood, dandelions are not weeds. They are magical toys, provided by God, to wish upon and run with. Clover is jewelry. The little girl perfected the art of making a clover bracelet, and made one for God. Before suppertime, she placed it on a low branch of a little tree. She knelt and prayed, telling God to please take it; it was made just for him. Early the next morning, she ran outside hoping it was gone. She stared at it with tears in her eyes. To this day, she remembers the disappointment she felt."

To me this demonstrates the difference between the immature and mature conception of God. The child expects instant, visible results. The mature person knows that spiritual results come from odd, unexpected directions, and tend to look like 'coincidences' or odd things that just 'somehow happened' at odds of thousands to one.

Answers can be very subtle – one reason some people say they do not even exist. How we receive our answers seems to be highly individual. It is somewhat similar to the private vocabulary of jokes and catch-phrases that lovers and very old friends have together, the kind of dialogue that can go on right in front of others without anyone being the wiser.

Some people say they learn to 'hear' a small voice inside of them, or a 'gut feeling' that seems to always be right. Some people feel they get definite replies in the form of sudden, unexpected events or omens. Some people say things 'just happen' – things so improbable that they cannot be easily explained.

It is hard to get people to talk about this. Julia Cameron, author of <u>The Artist's Way</u>, calls it 'synchronicity.' In <u>Conversations with God</u>, Neal Walsh's protagonist Voice explains to him that messages are being sent to us constantly in the form of outside events and cues. (When you hear a song on the radio that suddenly seems to directly address your private issue, it probably does.) Even Freud said there was no such thing as an accident, though he meant that rather differently. It is rather like dream symbols, in which the meanings are not fixed and not universal. They can be interpreted correctly only by the dreamer.

Sally, a young Bipolar student and painter, was the only one of my subjects who tried to put this synchronicity, the connivance of outside events to help us, into words.

> "I don't see coincidences any more, I see
> that those are natural happenings…I think God
> is an It. I think God is everything. I think that's
> kind of like the Hindu perspective – God is in

everything…you can't really see it, but you can experience it, you can feel it.

"Like, [I'm thinking] 'Gosh, how am I going to surmount all these thoughts going through my head? I feel so Depressed, I feel so crazy, I can't sleep, I'm so tired (sigh)'…I'm trying to make it happen, I'm trying to understand, or know God's hand in something, and it'll kind of run away from me? But if I just say, 'Fine, I'm not going to try to figure this out.' I just go about my business trusting that I'll get it, it always comes to me. I feel like, 'Oh!' I connect the dots. It just seems obvious.

"Things happen like that all the time…if I'm not seeing it, I'm probably Depressed.

"It's such a part of my life now. It happens all the time…I know I'll always be saved in the nick of time. In time, or just in the nick of time…You've just got to look for it when you're feeling lost and alone…if you can't find it, just surrender and it will happen.

"But you know, things happen like that all the time."

I find that when I am following this kind of spiritual guidance, my life starts going smoothly. I have heard people in Twelve-Step meetings say they get negative reinforcement: things go <u>wrong,</u> over and over, until they finally get the message that they must change their approach. However it happens, it does seem to happen recognizably once we have learned to watch for answers with an open mind.

Shelley, a retired special education teacher from San Francisco, prays this way:

"How do I know when I get an answer? I feel it. Oh, I don't say, 'I need this.' I pray for other people. And I see the results. When I see the results happen in other people then I know that it's come. It's happened.

"I prayed for my daughter so much when she was a methamphetamine addict. 'Please, please, God' – 'Cause you know, all your teeth fall out when you're thirty. You know, methamphetamine is one of the worst drugs we've got out now in our nation. And people manufacturing it – oh! Oh.

"Oh! And I used to do it so much! I lost my bottom little teeth. I'm going to have to wear a plate in my mouth at this young age, I mean it's crazy. Crazy, man.

"I thank God all the time. But I always want other people – I want [my help to go] *out* – I want it to be outwardly directed. I've given lots of freebies and I like doing that. It makes my soul sort of open up.

"I feel like I have a buddy, and maybe He can help, He, She, It...Them? It? Goddess? Whatever-have-you. I'm not sure. This entity that's outside of myself. I know I have problems, oh boy, I've got problems, but I know [it] when I feel it, the change."

How does all this relate to mental illness?
Well, for one thing, we need the help. We need the hope. It is my experience that prayer will not cure my condition; but it reminds me that I was not just crippled and then *abandoned*.
And some prayers are simply answered 'No.'

Then again, there are schools of thought that say I am wrong about that. Neal Walsh of <u>Conversations with God</u> says that we are merely praying the wrong way. His book claims that if you keep saying, "I need" or "I want," that is exactly what you get from the Universe: need and want. Lack. In other words, you will continue to want it and not get it. New Age theories tend to back this up. The idea is that if we use something more like an affirmation, such as *"Thank you* for giving me such and such," as if we had already received our request, we will find that it will come. This is probably what's behind 'The Law of Attraction' so heralded in the popular film, <u>The Secret</u>. Concentrate on what you want, not what you don't.

Since nobody is sure how prayer works, it behooves us to be at least somewhat open to such ideas. We really don't know enough about the universe, or God, to say, "What a stupid idea." In my experience, a persistent prayer will invariably provoke some kind of answer.

We need someone or something on our side who does not have to be educated about our medical condition. Someone who understands and will not expect us to buck up, cheer up, chin up, cure ourselves, act like everyone else, or otherwise do the impossible.

There are definite limits to what prayer and the energy of thought can do, however. Can prayer help people who are sick? Probably. Can it get your friend to recover from advanced cancer? Probably not, especially if your friend doesn't believe so.

This is why 'positive thinking' does not always work. It can be very harmful to us to run into these 'fix it by thinking' people.

Eddie relates running into this attitude professionally:

> "So later, they [sent me] to the really modern, you know humanistic kinds [of psychologists]? And they were just like 'Well! It's all in your mind! You just LIKE to think of yourself as screwed up, and you just don't WANT to exercise or try hard.'

"They were just these 'positive thinking' people, I don't know how they got their PhD. And so, you should just go jogging and, kind of, stop being an idiot. It was Orange County, you understand, it was the early Eighties, and it was totally just kind of the Me Decade....And nobody was REALLY sick there....It was just that YOU would [not] pull your shit together; this mental illness thing was just a story that people made up because they were wussies. You know. They were wimps, and they needed some weakling-ass story. And the miserable cowards just need to be studs. And then they'll get over it.

"And so THAT was my diagnosis for, like, another couple years."

We don't have to explain things to our Higher Power. It already knows. It takes away some of the bitterness and despair when we are able to trust that we are absolutely understood. Even if we can't be 'fixed', there is an awful lot we can pray for to improve our lives.

What to Pray For

Anything you want, of course. You are not going to hurt God's feelings by telling Him/Her/It what you really want.

This is my experience: chances are, if you pray for something long and intensely enough, you will get it. Or something like it. In my opinion, few prayers are ever truly and finally answered 'No.'

Jesus once said:

"If any of you has a friend, and goes to him in the middle of the night and says, 'Lend me three loaves, my dear fellow, for a friend of mine has just arrived after a journey and I have no food to put in front of him;' and then he answers from inside the house: 'Don't bother me with your troubles. The front door is locked and my children and I have gone to bed. I simply cannot get up now and give you anything!' Yet, I tell you, that even if he won't get up and give him what he wants simply because he is his friend, yet if he persists, he will rouse himself and give him everything he needs. And so I tell you, ask and it will be given you, search and you will find, knock and the door will be opened to you. The one who asks will always receive; the one who is searching will always find, and the door is opened to the man who knocks." (Luke 11:5, Phillips Version).

There is a catch to this secret, though. I would strongly advise you don't use it.

Why? Because what we want is not always smart. What we long for is often quite bad for us. When we want something too much, and our Power refuses it to us, over and over, it usually means that what we are asking for is something that will really hurt us.

I ought to know. That's how I got my first husband.

It's not an edifying story. I picked up this guy at the theater, see...he was handsome and shy and dark, just my type. He was listening and laughing quietly to himself at the jokes I made with the barristas. So I used the oldest trick in the world. It was a windy night, and I asked him to help light my cigarette. We got to talking. You know this story.

Well, about three months later I was desperately in love (oops!) and he started avoiding me. It turned out he needed a green card, and he had a friend who was pregnant and had been abandoned by her lover, so they were going to get married and save each other. He was Iranian, you see. It was the time of the Khomeini regime, and the hostage crisis – anybody remember that? If you were an Iranian national, and you'd been living in America, you could get off the plane back in Iran and just disappear. Not a good time to go home. So he was marrying someone else.

I prayed and cried and screamed and prayed some more. I stopped eating and nearly stopped functioning. I went down to 90 pounds – food nauseated me. I even went so far as to stalk him, parking in the driveway opposite, late at night, and watching his window to see if he would walk by it. I had fantasies of making friends with the other woman and poisoning her tea. I don't even drink tea.

I kept praying, obsessively.

Well, don't you know, that woman's lover came back and claimed his child, and the marriage to my boyfriend was annulled and like an ass I said, 'Hey, if you need a green card, I'LL marry you. Just don't go marrying anyone else! '

And that's how, at age 20, I married a man who did not love me a bit. This started two years of cultural and emotional warfare that nearly killed me. I actually sat in our living room one day, looking out at a beautiful peach tree in bloom, and contemplated whether I should buy a gun. You know, to point at my head. To fire.

But you can't say I wasn't warned! God said 'no' and 'no' and 'no' until I starved myself down to 90 pounds; then he gave in. Which of us was right about my welfare and happiness?

This is basically the reason it's recommended to "pray only for our Higher Power's will and the ability to carry that will out." Not because we are small and unimportant and ought to Obey. No. It's because the Universe has plans for us that will ultimately feel better, work better, help us grow faster, and otherwise get the best long-term deal from our limited time on earth. No matter how it looks on paper, your plans are going to hurt worse and help you less than whatever God has planned. Honest.

So if you're really smart, that's the way to go.

An Odd Footnote

Eddie told me this little anecdote:

"I was once at a Hindu temple, and a priest was attempting to prepare a mixed Anglo-Indian couple for a formal Hindu wedding. And as such, the woman's dad was there having Hinduism explained to him.

"This particular priest said that he believed that an important part of religious life for him was having desires to bring before the gods.

"So, far from saying our desires should be repressed, he seemed to relish the idea of – so to speak – giving the gods a chance to prove themselves; and had we no desires, it would be hard to see how they could do this."

If the whole idea of prayer leaves you cold

Well, that's fine. But you probably pray anyway and just don't know it.

Do you do affirmations? Do you visualize the effects you want to achieve? Do you daydream, hard and long, about the kind of life you are looking for? Those are prayers, actually. It's all thought energy.

Synchronicity is something most people experience. You start thinking about a new idea, and suddenly you meet an authority in the field, or run into a book on it. You decide you want to fly somewhere, and suddenly there is a price war for fares to that country. Odd helping hands out of left field. Timing that is just *too* good. I've lived long enough, and seen enough of this, to stop believing in coincidence. (Freud didn't either, by the way).

Because the thing we forget – I don't know why – is that the motive power that created the cosmos millions of years ago does not require human language (which is only a few thousands of years old, anyway) to know what we need.

Thoughts are energy, and energy goes straight to the divine heart of things.

As for getting guidance back from a Force that may be vague to you: women call it 'intuition.' Men call it a 'gut feeling' or a 'hunch.' The bible calls it a 'still, small voice.'

Seriously now, if you think back, how often was that little voice wrong?

Possible Side Effects

This is a phrase you've probably heard a lot, every time something new gets prescribed for you. But for once, the side effects are all good.

The greatest boon of the Third Step is what happens in our minds. When we let go of results, the relief is stupendous.

For the PASC, sometimes even basic needs are hard to meet. Having a place to live. Medicine. An income. People to help you, to care. Just filling out all the forms demanded by government agencies is enough to challenge anyone!

The Twelve-Step difference is that once you've filled out those forms, instead of waiting on pins and needles for the next six weeks, you can forget them. Either your request will be approved, or it won't. Your Higher Power will decide. *And if the Power says 'no,' you can be absolutely certain that something better is in store for you.*

This takes away an immense load of worry and frantically looking for a solution – none of which is especially good for us. Living in the moment is extra-important for special chemistry people, because we have even less control than the average person over what happens next (that is, other people get to *think* they have more control!).

My experience is that on days when I work a sincere Third Step, I actually may need less medicine. My symptoms decrease as I relax. I become happier, more efficient, more "plugged in" to reality. In other words, *living by the Third Step makes me more sane.* Measurably. Visibly.

If Anxiety is your problem, this Step is the single best thing you can do for yourself.

I believe it can do the same for many of us – if we are willing.

Outer Tips to Inner Peace

Strategy 3: Environmental Cues

I first wrote this section with the assumption that all special chemistry people need as calm and serene an environment as possible. I gave a lot of tips for how to achieve that, especially on a budget.

But then I realized I had missed the point.

What we need as PASC patients is *some place to feel safe.*

Safe means different things to different people. Safe *may* mean calm and serene and pretty. But it may not. Maybe 'safe' to you means a place where you can just be your sloppy self. Where you can drop anything on the floor, and not pick it up for a week or a month, and no one will nag you. Maybe 'safe' means having furniture that you never have to worry about staining or tearing because it is already completely destroyed. Maybe 'safe' means it is small and dark like a womb. Maybe 'safe' means all your favorite clutter around you, and never mind what it looks like or if it is organized. I knew a man who felt happy and safe only if he was surrounded by pictures of naked women cut out of magazines. They were taped all over his wall. Hey, it worked for him!

All of this is fine.

What I want us to aim for, in PASC condition, is a place – no matter how small, or in what horrible neighborhood – that when you close the door makes you breathe a sigh of relief. The place to run to when you are losing it and MUST get away. A place where it's OK to be yourself, no matter how strange that self may be. That is the goal.

However you accomplish that is fine. By the way, if you *are* in the horrible neighborhood, maybe 'safe' means having a lot of locks on the door and almost never going out. In that case, it is especially important you feel good about your space, because you will spend a *lot* of time there.

If you are not a clean or organized person, so what? Clean and organized is no proof of sanity, no matter what your mother told you.

There are only two things I really advise you to keep organized: your pills, and any paperwork about your condition.

No, your pills don't need to be in neat little rows on a rattan tray. But they need to be always in the same place, where you can get to them absolutely without thinking, even if you are seeing monsters (or whatever). You need to be organized enough that you NEVER RUN OUT. I can't think of anything more important than that. My method is just to turn the bottle upside down on the nightstand when the number of pills in it gets low. That way, first thing in the morning I notice it and call the pharmacy.

And your paperwork? That can be really simple. Just have any old box with a folder in it for each subject you need to keep track of: for example, one for Medicare, one for your Psychiatrist, and one for welfare benefits (or whatever services or income you receive). Whatever the latest paper is relating to that subject, put it inside the folder *in front of all the older papers.* If the most recent thing is on top, you can always find it in a hurry. You don't have to dig or look for dates or any of that. Just keep the stupid old box in the same old place all the time, so you can always throw something right into it, and always pull something right out of it. Easy. This basic organization is so important I think I may repeat myself later.

Oh, and one more thing. It is critical to have a phone number (or numbers, if you like) right by the phone for psychiatric emergencies. Taped on is a good idea if you only use a cell. If you are going critical in your head, or you need a hospital or doctor *right now,* you are not going to be in any shape to page through the phone book looking for help. If you can't even see straight right that minute, you can just say, "It's taped on the phone!" to whoever's around.

That said, here are my handy-dandy tips for those of you after a little visible serenity in your surroundings.

Depending on your condition, your surroundings can make a great difference to your level of peace and comfort.

Pablo, who is Obsessive-Compulsive, described this at length to me.

> "The phobias can be so...disabilitating [sic] that I couldn't function. You couldn't leave the house because you're afraid of being contaminated. And the ultimate fear is you will die. You're going to be poisoned by something, and you're going to *die* from it. So you just don't go out...

> "I'm always on edge just a little bit. So when you're with people or a situation where you feel comfortable, then things are all right – in the sense you don't get scared, you don't get frightened by things. The Obsessive behavior will tone down. The Obsessive behavior is more of a warding off – of trying to keep imagined threats away from you, whether it's germs on a doorknob or some axe-murderer waiting outside your door...The safety makes a *big* difference...

> "Or even the décor of a house. It is so sensitive. Of course, if you're in your own place you can make your own décor...Just a sense of – I can look around this room for example – just a sense of artistic arrangement...whoever arranged these candles...That brings a kind of serenity, than if they were just helter-skelter and all different...see, there is an arrangement. That has a kind of peaceful effect. And it's a very subtle thing. It's subtle. But it's there, and it's important. A lot of people pay no attention to that. I mean, if I walk into someone's home, which is just totally filled with clutter – because that's the way they might like to live –

I can hardly spend 15 minutes there before I've got to get out!

    "...Let's give you another example. I go to a park that has nicely mowed grass and it's manicured. And then you see someone's left some trash there. Well, immediately that is a violation to me against the mood that is *supposed* to be there. And I'm inclined, I'll go over and pick it up and put it, you know – to correct that because it just comes in and jars you up. Now I think the average person, it doesn't bother them. But this is a problem.

    "...Once I went to visit some people's property that was really very isolated back in the Mendocino National Forest area where they had bought some property. Totally in the sticks. Went there, and they weren't there, I was there by myself. Just enjoying this, and then guess what broke that serenity? A jet plane flying overhead. I thought to myself, 'If I had a gun I'd shoot it down!' Because it just totally broke apart that whole scene. And destroyed it. But there's that sensitivity again.

    "...Because when you're fighting those things that trouble you in the environment and that irritate you all the time, and they're continuous, and you have no way to change it, then it just has – it's harder to dig out of that. That's the only way I could put it."

Some sense of order can be useful to our mental health. This is the best reason for things like doing laundry and keeping the room clean. Peace and quiet can be important, too – but also hard to achieve.

Many PASC people can't work at all and live on the dole. They may have no choice about where they live. Whatever hotel is subsidized by their county is where they end up – often in one room with no kitchen and a window on the airshaft.

One of the simplest things to do for yourself is surround yourself with the right colors. People respond profoundly to the colors around them. There is a New Age practice called Aura-soma wherein a client picks their 3 favorite bottles from a brilliant-hued array of 100. By analyzing the shades they pick, a trained practitioner can tell with startling accuracy just who this person is and what issues they are facing in their lives. That is how connected we are to the colors we like and dislike.

It costs next to nothing to paint a room, or even just one wall, in your favorite shade. If you're not allowed to paint, you can hang a swag of fabric in the right hue, or posters – showing anything at all – in a color that makes you smile. When you pick up a quilt from the Goodwill, it doesn't cost a thing to pick the color that you like, not the dull 'practical' one. A piece of cloth thrown over your nightstand; shiny rocks or pieces of coral arranged on your desk; there are dozens of ways to bring happy, soothing colors into your space. Cover that airshaft with a horizontal string of beads, or ribbons, or cheerful gauzy curtains. Try cheap pillows to make that saggy twin bed into a comfy couch.

This is the single best tip for the low-budget wardrobe, too. An old T-shirt *in the right color* can make you look as good as a designer shirt in the wrong one. Each one of us has a set of colors that make our face and eyes and hair look radiant and alive, and also colors that drain us to a deathly hue. And think about how depressing the dull darkness of winter can be. Part of that is absence of color.

Go to the library and find one of the dozens of beauty or cosmetic or fashion books that will tell you what your best personal colors are. (Guys, just tell the librarian the book is for your sister, and take it home in a brown paper bag!)

If you work, and have to dress conservatively, there is nothing stopping you from having the right color striped subtly into your tweed suit. You will look better, but no one will know why. Ties and scarves work, too.

For the adventurous: be aware that if you dye your hair, your whole color wheel might change. Different things look good on a redhead than on a blonde or brunette.

Color is an emotional tool. Use it in your favor.

Music to Your Ears

Music can reach anyone. It is a great mood-changer and brain-distracter. Depression can get a lift, Mania and Anxiety can be temporarily soothed, and inner voices can be partially drowned out or distracted. This is one place I'd advise you to indulge.

Whatever style you like is fine, but fit it to your needs. If you are thinking suicide, don't put on a Mahler symphony. If you are scared to walk out in your neighborhood, gangsta rap may not be your best choice. That's why it's good to collect different kinds and genres. Explore a little. You can probably afford to try a strange new piece of music via LP or cassette tape, if your budget doesn't run to CD's and iPods.

If all else fails, twiddle the dials of a cheap radio.

There are other soothing noises you can put in your environment. Wind chimes of all kinds are one idea – wood, bamboo, glass, ceramic, different kinds of metal in different thicknesses. You don't need a real wind – just touch them to make a sweet or slithery sound.

There are also some really glorious nature CDs out now, as well as meditation and relaxation tapes. The sound of a forest or ocean may be just what you need.

My favorite is a desktop waterfall. I have an elegant little fake-granite number on my desk that I picked up for ten bucks on eBay. It helps to have that rippling in the background. Especially when I'm adding up all the (red!) numbers in my checkbook.

Sometimes silence is best, of course. But we often live too close together these days. Constant noise is the curse of modern existence. If your walls are thin and the neighbors are loud, try a Sound Soother or other white-noise machine. Using one tends to cut off all but the worst random noise, if placed between you and the source. Some machines have sound choices such as the ocean. Psychologists sometimes use them to soundproof their offices so outsiders can't hear confidential talks, another advantage to consider. These machines can be inexpensive, too – or ask for one as a birthday or holiday gift.

This is also another place that fountains can help.

The Best Sound of All

When you're lonely and unhappy, the best sound is the voice of someone who cares. Use your telephone!

Shanna, when I asked her for the one piece of advice she'd give to other PASC people, said, "Don't hold it in to the extent where you're going to explode. Just hold it in long enough to talk to somebody. Here is what I have to do still, even on my medicine."

Be judicious, lest you wear one person out too much. Call different people on different days. After (or before!) you've unloaded, ask them how *they're* doing – and show interest in the answers. You're going to need your friends as never before. Treat them well. Be sure they get something from you besides the blues.

Some things you just can't say to the average person living the Average American Life, though. It doesn't compute. This is where Twelve-Step meetings come in. Not only can you talk and listen for tips at meetings, you are encouraged to *take phone numbers*. These people understand serious problems. They know what they're getting into.

Not all Twelve-Step groups are willing (or able) to handle special chemistry issues. The ones that deal with human relationships can be helpful. Your best bet is probably your local Emotions Anonymous meeting. Their problems may not be strictly PASC related, but they are emotional and psychological. You may even choose a mentor (called a Sponsor) to help you work through the Twelve Steps.

You will meet, and should cultivate, other PASC persons who are more or less functional. There are conversations we cannot have with outsiders. I remember a long discussion with other hospital patients about methods of suicide they'd considered, and the pros and cons of each. No way could you have this conversation with average people. They would be horrified and try to change the subject. But we all got a lot of relief from it, and there were even some good belly laughs. This is valuable. You can't get it anywhere else.

Your most complex stuff, of course, should be shared in therapy. Therapy is a must for most of the PASC, at least until they have been stabilized on their medicines for a while. Don't stop until you have learned a good handful of techniques to deal with your most common patterns of behavior. Some therapists are familiar with the Twelve Steps, which can be helpful. In any case, therapy is like an automatic and continuing Fifth Step – a very good idea, as we will see.

Studies have shown that therapy and medicine are about equally productive in producing PASC improvement. Statistically, people get the best results if they hammer at it from both sides.

My other tip is to cultivate about equal numbers of PASC and 'normal' friends, to keep an even perspective. The world consists of both, and your life should, too.

As Pablo said to me: "If you can keep those positive connections going, meaningful for you, you won't trip and fall down."

PART THREE:

SHAME ON WHOM?

Now I'm not looking for Absolution
Peace of mind after what I've been through
and before you come to any conclusion
try walking in my shoes...
You'd stumble in my footsteps
you'd keep the same appointments I've kept
if you tried walking in my shoes
Try walking in my shoes
--Depeche Mode

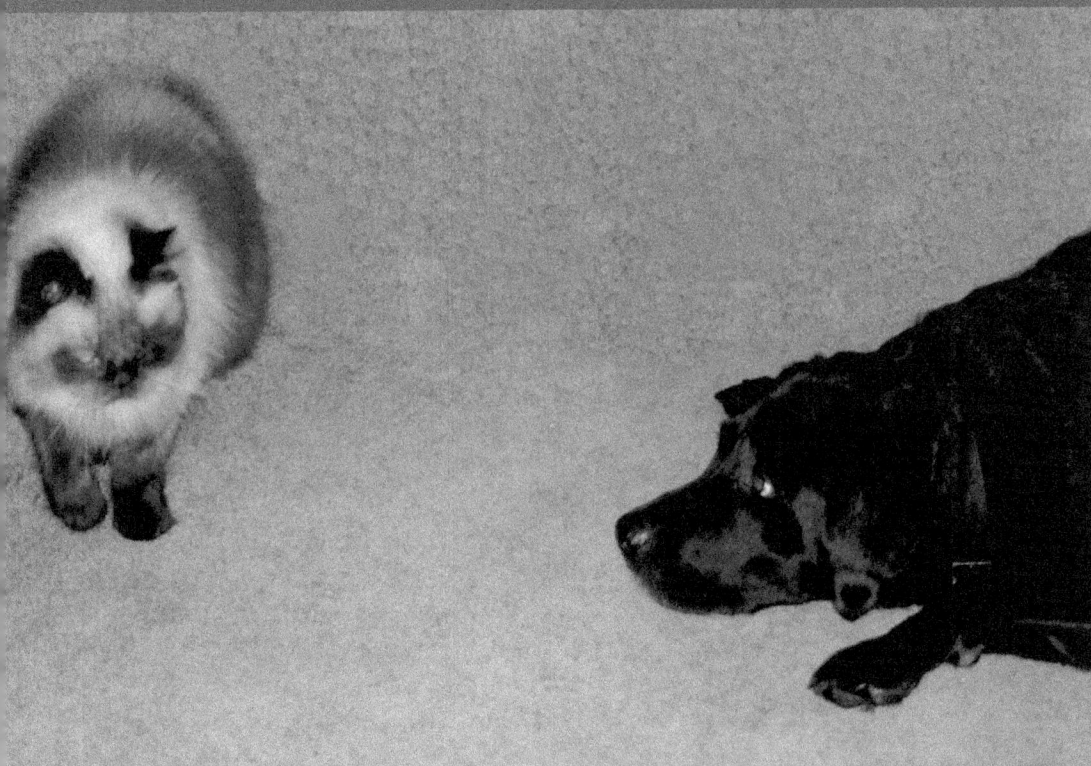

STEP FOUR

Look at Who You Are

"Made a searching and fearless
moral inventory of ourselves."
-- adapted from the Twelve Steps of AA

STEP FOUR

Taking inventory of yourself is challenging. It occurs to me you might not want to do this. Few people do.

But this is part of finding your new identity after a diagnosis. Who are you now? What's right and wrong about you? What do you have left if your brain isn't working for you? We need to know what raw materials we're working with, because once a person is labeled 'crazy,' the rules change.
An inventory is a lot like exercise. Most of us don't look forward to it, but we feel great afterwards.

In the 'Big Book' and among Twelve-Step followers, sometimes a lot of energy gets expended on the 'how' of inventories. It doesn't matter how. If you're the detail type, you can do a chronological scan of your life. Or you can make a list of incidents where you were not happy with your own behavior. If you feel you already know yourself pretty well, start listing your characteristics on a 'pro' and 'con' sheet and see where it takes you. You can write it all out, or if writing doesn't work for you, you can record it all in a normal, conversational voice on a tape recorder. Listening to it later can be revealing. Sometimes your tone of voice will tell you more than the words. *Oops, sounds like I don't believe what I just said!*

It doesn't really matter how you do it. What matters is that you take your own inventory, not anybody else's, and that you use your own standards of what's moral. This is not an ethics test. You are looking for areas where you are disappointed in yourself, not where others are unhappy.

The 'Big Book' uses lots of space on how to take your own inventory, and it's worth reading. In summary, the book says that buried in every incident where somebody hurt or angered or disappointed you, there is a way in which you hurt or angered or disappointed yourself. These are your vulnerabilities. Learning to sweep your own side of the street is an important part of the inventory.

If you are still in too much pain and resentment to do this right now, that's OK. That's what therapy is for. Unburden yourself of as much pain as you can, and then come back to this Step. There's no hurry.

What you are looking for here is not pages and pages of 'times I did things wrong,' but for patterns. Never mind all those bastards you dated – what is it in you that keeps picking those kinds of partners? Never mind whose fault all those fights were, or what they said to you – what is it about you that gets you into fights? This is where the real insights come in. (You could ask your best friend to tell you, but be ready to be shocked and dismayed. You asked.)

If you don't see the reasons for your patterns right away, don't worry. That is another thing therapy is good for. It can take a long time to dig out some of the sneaky stuff we do to ourselves. You don't have to figure it all out today. Just notice that something is happening over and over, and leave a mental note to look at it later.

Be clear on one thing, though: we are talking about your *character* here, not your *disease*.

Take your time. Be thorough and searching, as the Step says.

I will say that being 'fearless' about it is nothing I've ever accomplished. I do try to remember, however, that a Higher Power made me as I am, and can work with me in any condition. It's not as if S/He didn't already know.

Trouble seeing ourselves clearly is not a special prerogative of the psychotic. Everybody has a natural resistance to seeing personal flaws exactly as they are. We prefer to glamorize them, or justify them, or dramatize them. Something that will turn them into proofs of eccentric genius, or endearing quirks. Anything other than what they are, which is yucky personal traits.

But you may have done this before. Whether we want them or not, we all sometimes have moments of truth. We are arguing with someone ferociously, for instance, and they say something that snaps into our head: 'You know, she's right. I *am* impatient and stubborn'. Or we do something with such bad consequences that we *know* it was stupid. Nobody has to tell us (although they probably will). We have moments of truth when we've hurt somebody beyond ever being forgiven. Or the moment we admitted we really were alcoholics or addicts, if that's our history.

We've already had one moment of unwelcome clarity when we understood there was something wrong with our brain.

So if we've have lived through that, we are in a good position to do a Fourth Step. In comparison, it might even be easy.

Psychological Step Four

The main question is how the Fourth Step applies to being PASC.

Here is the key: *SYMPTOMS ARE NOT MORAL FAILINGS.*

We might, in the beginning, be tempted to harrow ourselves over all our most bizarre and inappropriate behaviors. That is a false lead. We are not looking for out-of-control incidents right now. We will get to that, but it does not become practical and important until Step Eight. In the meanwhile, if those incidents bother you, make a list and set it aside. Clear your mind for today's serious work.

Now ask yourself this question: What has mental illness added to your personality?

The easiest flaw to detect is failure to deal with the facts.

Non-Compliance

This is a term used to indicate a pattern of denying one's illness and refusing to take medication.

Maybe you do take meds. Sometimes. But then you feel better, so you figure you only needed them for a little while but not anymore. And you stop. Or you break your appointment with your therapist or psychiatrist. Because after all, you weren't that sick in the first place, were you? Can't people see how much you've improved? That's it, folks – I'm cured! All gone.

You may be okay for a while, but the disease has not gone away.

Non-compliance is extra troublesome with dual-diagnosis patients. The doctors don't know why, but I do. We're good at denial. We've had a lot of practice, with our booze and our drugs and our other nasty little obsessions.

Face reality. You have what you have. You are what you are. Take your medicine.

About Medicine

Speaking of medical matters, this is as good a time as any to dispose of a major bugbear.

Taking prescribed psychiatric medication is NOT 'substance abuse.'

This is a point that confuses a lot of sincere, innocent people, and can cause a lot of misplaced guilt. Some recovering people have even been talked into discontinuing treatment. This is wrong. It is unnecessary. It is ignorant and interfering, to be blunt. And it isn't even 'good program,' as working on the Steps successfully is called.

> "Some of us have had to cope with Depressions that can be suicidal; Schizophrenia that sometimes requires hospitalization; Manic Depression; and other mental and biological illness...some members have taken the position that no one in AA should take any medication...[but] just as it is wrong to enable or support any alcoholic to become re-addicted to any drug, it's equally wrong to deprive any alcoholic of medication which can alleviate or control other disabling and/or emotional problems."

- The AA Member: Medications and other Drugs

That's official program literature I'm quoting. So if someone tries to convince you not to take your medicine, forget it. I've seen people refuse medicine because 'God will cure you if you pray and believe'. They just get sicker. If someone talks to you like that, don't listen.

The major caution about meds is to take them
1) Only as prescribed
2) Only the minimum needed.

After all, some of us are addicts; there's always the temptation to pop a little extra to see if it works better! Don't. Psychiatric drugs are potent, and careless use can be toxic or even fatal.

One other major caution. Be sure that the person prescribing for you knows that you have a history of substance abuse, if you do. That way they can steer clear of anything that might cause you problems, and offer a substitute. And if you suffer from suicidal impulses, your doctor must know that, too. You can be given less dangerous meds, or arrange for someone neutral to dole out your daily dose to you.

Let's suppose denial is not one of our faults at present, and we are doing all we can to stay well. What other defects are we liable to? How have you changed since you developed special chemistry?

What I am going to list in the following pages are weak spots I have found in myself. I offer them in the hope that they will jog your self-examination, even if your particular flaws are nothing like mine.

I'm Too Sick

Have you ever avoided something you just didn't want to do by claiming you were too ill? Or blamed your disease for a behavior that it was in your power to change? Have you tried to get pity or favors or attention because of your condition? I know these are not pretty questions. But in the not so pretty real world, I have done these things a time or two. It's all too easy to abuse the 'I'm sick' excuse. The danger in this is that when you

really need help, people might be tired of helping you, or feel
that you're crying wolf, and ignore you when you need them
most.

Poor Me

When I was first diagnosed, I asked my therapist what
my greatest risk would be. I expected some spectacular answer,
like, 'don't eat beef or you'll run over a cliff'...instead she looked
me straight in the face and said, "Self-pity".
Busted.
Even if I didn't try to make others sorry for me, I often
waddled in neck-deep pity for my poor little damaged self.
No one can blame us for sometimes feeling pretty sorry
about this mess we didn't ask for. Sometimes. But beyond that,
it's like poking an infected tooth. Why do it? Do you like pain?
For instance, sometimes I get very boo-hooey over the
American Dream as portrayed on TV. I'll never meet that
standard – I can't work enough to earn that salary. And it's not
my fault! And it's not fair! Why can't I have fashionable clothing
and a house in a ritzy residential area? Why can't I have a car
that reminds me of a panther and streaks along curvy shore
roads?
I have special trouble with this whenever I hit a decade
birthday. I think, 'I should have this by now. Ordinary people
do. Ordinary people can work 40 hours a week. They can learn
new skills and switch careers if they want to. Ordinary people
finish school by the time they're 30 and find a partner without
worrying about when to betray their Dark Secret.'
Well, OK, all these things may be true (notice I said *may*
be). I may have spent 30 years learning to live with my disease
while other people were using that time in other ways. And
occasionally this does make me sad.
But is it true that I am deprived?
First of all, I have never hankered after the forty-hour
week and settled career. I have always wanted to be a writer. So
the chances are I would not have spent those years climbing the
corporate ladder even were I free to do so.

Secondly - and you already know this - the advertising machinery of this country is not a trustworthy measure of what we 'should' be, or by what age we 'should' be there. Advertising is to make people want the product, buy the product, make the company some profit, and keep the good old economy going. That is its purpose. Not your purpose. Not necessarily in your best interests at all.

Thirdly, what is the good of thinking this way? Why moan about what I've missed? If I must look back, why not look at what I've achieved? As of this writing, I am in my 17th year of recovery[1]. I am no longer afraid to go out in public, or afraid that if I don't watch out I'll do something awful to the ones I love. I have a part-time job, one that I can believe in. I have people in my life whom I respect and love, and they respect and love me in return. Would I really trade that in for a Lexus?

Fourthly, and most importantly, this self-pity is based on a false premise. It assumes that everyone without my disease is happy and normal. Or at most, they have only minor problems that don't stack up against mine.

It's just an illusion. The longer I live, the more I find that everyone has some burden. Some of those burdens are incredibly awful. Just because you can't see the crack doesn't mean somebody's not broken. We have not been specially picked out for grief and suffering. The human race is a sort of Special Olympics, and everyone gets a suitable handicap. This is ours.

Isolation

There has long been a warning in rehabilitation circles that says: "Don't get too hungry, angry, lonely, or tired: H.A.L.T." Very good advice.

---

[1] By the time I finished this book, I had reached 20 years sober, and married a wonderful man. I even have my house in the suburbs, by God! So you never know.

I'd like to expand on the "lonely" part. I would include isolation, which covers a lot more ground than mere loneliness. Isolation suggests alienation, being shut out, different, unable to communicate or even attempt a connection. Being too far away psychically or physically for anyone to reach.

Don't confuse isolation with solitude. Solitude can be splendid, if voluntary, and is a great healing tool when the world becomes too overwhelming. Withdrawing to put our heads back together can be an absolute necessity at times. Solitude is useful for resting, planning, dreaming, and thinking things through. Or even picking our nose, if we want to (hey, if nobody's looking...!).

Isolation, on the other hand, can be downright dangerous for the PASC. We already have an overdeveloped sense of 'difference.' We already tend to huddle alone with our symptoms and substances. What happens if we get completely separated from the world? Suppose there's a sudden emergency, such as a psychotic break, or running out of medication or food and being unable to function enough to get more? And that's just the practical side. There are more psychological reasons than I can count for not isolating.

I do know that there are days when nothing else is possible. Don't think for a minute that I haven't gone through that (and probably will again). Days, or weeks, when staring at the wall all day is the best I can do. (Hey, at least my eyes are open. What more could anybody ask?)

However, when we are able to get up, we should do what we can to maintain contact with the outside world. If we can't talk, we can listen to the radio or watch TV for outside events and topics to think about (besides whether anybody would care if we died). If there's anything outside our window, we can look at it. If we're able to talk, but not leave the house, the best thing is to contact friends via telephone or computer. There have been long periods when this was my only social contact, and I am convinced that it saved my life once or twice.

If you're PASC, hanging around in your head too long without company can be dangerous.

If you can get dressed, if you feel strong enough to leave the house, do. There are things you can do without needing conversation. Sit in the local café or even a McDonald's near a street or intersection and watch all the other humans go by. Or go to a local garden or park and just walk around looking at the other living things. Is there a nearby lake, beach, trail, or forest? Even a grove of trees will do. It can help you reconnect with living things (and with your Higher Power) without demanding much from you but that you be there.

And when you're ready to talk again, be sure you pick the most accepting, understanding people you can. This is a vulnerable time. Don't set yourself up for rejection or indifference that will send you running back to your room.

Well, you get the idea. If you're gentle with yourself, and realistic about your ability to function, there are ways to touch the rest of the world without letting it eat you up.

I Don't Care

This attitude could be the 'hungry and tired' part of the acronym H.A.L.T. When we get sick enough, we just don't care about things anymore. We might just stop eating when food is exactly what we need.

Apathy is a common fault, including apathy about hygiene. It's not unusual for the Depressed to be unable to tell you when they had their last shower, or their last meal. It is important to take care of our bodies. When we don't care for ourselves, we're basically stating there's nothing there worth caring about. And then when people avoid the smelly person we've created, we think they don't care either. It is all a very defeating cycle.

Sometimes the inner world clamors for all our attention. It can seem to fill up the whole universe. There are occasions when not acting out our inner turmoil takes everything we've got. There are days when simply staying alive can be a moral victory.

Nevertheless, that draining mind does live in a body, and that body needs care. Not eating, or eating only unhealthy foods; not ever exercising or getting any fresh air; not sleeping or its converse, sleeping for days on end; all of these things can contribute to keeping you sick. Not just physically, but psychologically. (As you know, your chances for substance abuse go up, too.)

I'm not saying be perfect despite your agony. But try to do the minimum.

It's good to develop some regular daily routines that we do every day automatically. Then, when we get Depressed and all the juice runs out of us, we will still find ourselves going through the motions, just enough to keep us alive.

See that there is some food in the house (some of it vegetable). Our minds and our medicines will work better with fuel. Even if we feel awful, it is possible to go to the grocery store once a week and buy a few veggies, some fruits, and some meat (if you eat meat) or rice and beans.

If our problem is Depression, exercise will help us feel better. Even a little bit counts. One walk around the block is a great victory if we wish we were dead. If our problem is anger or Mania, exercise will help derail some of that way-out energy. If our medications are making us blow up to elephant size, exercise will help keep the weight-gain down. If Anxiety or insomnia keeps us awake, again, a good hard workout can use up our body enough that sleep will come more easily.

I don't mean to sound like your mother. I just know from experience that the physical shape I'm in contributes to the mental shape I'm in. It can affect the course of our recovery and/or the severity of our symptoms. A body that is well-fed and well worked will assist us in being calmer, more balanced, and more resourceful.

If all that's just too much, the answer is to get someone else to help us. They can shop for us, for instance, or come to our house to get us when it's time to go to the gym. It's hard to ask, but it's one of the things the Twelve-Step program teaches – we must reach out. We can't afford to be completely alone.

Anger

This is the last subject using the H.A.L.T. acronym.

Anger is inevitable. If we have a shred of self-respect, we are going to get mad at what is happening to us sometimes. The main thing is to discharge it safely.

We can try serious physical work. Rearrange all the furniture in the house. Or work out, as suggested above. We can try talking to friends, with the caveat that we don't too often use the same people for the same old complaint. A therapist is an ideal repository for anger. A diary is another good place. If writing is not your bag, try recording your furious feelings on tape. Then play it back later when you're cooler. I've learned some interesting things about myself that way. The words may lie, but the tone of voice doesn't.

Some people get lots of mileage out of minor violence – throwing rocks at the fence, or beating on pillows, or crashing cheap old porcelain plates from Goodwill. Whatever works, as long as no one gets hurt.

The main thing to remember is that anger is blind. It pushes us just that much further toward the irrational. We can't afford that. Find a way to dissipate it.

Resentment and Jealousy

It goes (almost) without saying that the PASC are in danger if they carry such feelings around. If we are working this Step by the Big Book model, we might try looking at these resentments in the way prescribed there.

We may resent our doctors, who don't seem to listen. What about our pharmacists, who can't ever seem to fill our prescriptions in time? Or who always run out of our brand just when we're empty? Or our insurance companies – now there's a good one! Do you hate the sour-faced nurse on the D Ward? The whole hospital? The people who say if you would just (fill in the blank) you would be all better? Do you resent the whole 'normie' world?

We may have good reasons for all of those resentments. In fact, I'm sure we do. The state of the PASC could stand a lot of improvement, to say no more. But holding on to these feelings will only help our illness, not us. Living one day at a time means letting go of past grievances. It means trusting our Higher Power for the outcome – yes, even of that stack of papers we turned in to Medicaid two months ago! Stop trying to control things. The relaxation that ensues may even help with your symptoms. Take a deep breath here and go back to Step Three.

Sense Of Entitlement

There are some people – I'm sure you've met some – who feel that the whole world owes them something. They are the ones who make 32 clients wait behind them in line while their (non)problem is solved.

Maybe they want extra time at the computer, because they are too poor to afford their own, or too sick. Or maybe they are too rich or important! Or maybe they are too famous or beautiful to be bothered with the likes of us. These are the people that demand extra time and attention everywhere they go, and give nothing back, not even thanks. The world *owes* it to them. They feel entitled.

Do not become one of these people!

It is a temptation one must fight. Yes, we have a special condition; it is very hard, and sometimes we need extra help. There is a time to ask for it pleasantly and politely. But we must realize that others have a right to say 'no' to us.

It's not infrequent that I get harangued for money in the local city. I don't ignore these people, I simply say, "Hey, I'm on Disability; I don't' have any money either. Good luck." You should see the surprised looks I get. They are so busy with their own drama it never occurs to them that someone else might have similar problems.

We are not the only ones with horrible challenges, even though others may appear to be doing better. That woman you saw with the furs and diamonds may have a husband who is dying from leukemia. That handsome bachelor may have lost a wife and two children to a fire. That guy with the well-controlled, razor-sharp mind may be afflicted with muscular dystrophy. We may think the worst thing is not to have control of our minds. But he could justifiably think that a great mind is no compensation when carried around in a rotting body.

Let me tell you a little story. I knew a fellow – let's call him Brandon – who was dying of alcohol abuse. This is sad, and it's understandable that he gave up his apartment and went to live with his family for his remaining time.

But Brandon felt entitled. He did not tell his family he was coming; he just got on a plane and arrived. He left behind a full apartment and even a dog. He expected his family to go 2,000 miles and pack it all up for him and bring it back to him; he didn't even give them money for the trip or the shipping.

His family did not have lots of money. They decided to do this for him, but they could only afford to rent a very small car, and take only what was important, clothes and personal effects. They did not take every piece of paper they saw, for instance. Doesn't everybody have lots of waste paper in their household, old letters, laundry lists, ideas and phone numbers scribbled down that they never get to? His family didn't keep the scattered papers.

They did the whole job, drove 2,000 miles twice for him.

For the rest of his life, Brandon complained that his family had viciously thrown out his poems. His family thought they were grocery lists.

Granted, it would be a bitter blow to me if I ever lost my poem collection. But whose job was it, really, to salvage and move those papers? Brandon lost his poems, and everybody lost his goodwill, because Brandon felt *entitled* to have everyone work for him for free.

Please, please, don't become 'one of those people.' Understand that everybody has tests and challenges in life.

A Word About Reasonable Accommodation

You have probably heard about the Americans with Disabilities Act, and are vaguely aware that you have some rights. This is true. However, getting them applied to your case can be another story. There is a website that will tell you what kind of reasonable accommodations you are entitled to in the workplace (http://www.bu.edu/cpr/reasaccom/). But you will find that not all places honor them, and that you may not have a job if you insist on them. Whether you take this to court is up to you. I have great respect for those who do, and they do us all a favor.

But on the whole, you will find that the working world is not going to make exceptions for you – not for long, anyhow. You may have a supervisor who understands for a couple of years – but what do you do when that supervisor moves on or moves up?

I am not saying don't pursue your rights. I'm just saying, don't expect them to be handed to you. Eddie describes his work experience wryly:

> "My bosses aren't obligated to give me a raise 'cause I'm in pain. Our culture is that businessmen just have *no* moral duty…So in other words, it would be like asking an executioner not to chop off heads. He's an executioner. You could talk with him about anything. I suppose you could ask him not to cut off heads; but that's unfair, because he's an executioner.
>
> "…Kind of a waste of time…And it's *unfair*, because he's an executioner. Businessmen *are* henchmen. They're criminals. And they're *sanctioned*. Like, what they do, that is morally criminal, is legal. So in other words, we've said to them as a group, 'Business men are *exempt* from ethics.'
>
> "So you can't say, 'You're my boss, and I work with you every day and we care about each other, so of course, you're obligated to attempt to see to my needs.' You could even say that and he would say (snort, snigger) 'I gotta go now.' He wouldn't even fire you because it's so absurd it wouldn't even be

threatening...And the next day he'd go, 'Hi, there. Have a good day.'

"They're free to hear whatever, since it's in advance admitted that they have no obligation. So as a result, oddly...I mean, they have a little resistance at first because they like me, and they find it hard to believe that this likeable of a guy really has this magnitude of a problem, but once I make it simply clear to them with evidence, then they're just like, 'Wow,' or whatever. 'Whoa. Huh. See you tomorrow.' (laughter) And the next day, 'Let's go.'"

Et Cetera

Briefly, here are some other things to look for in your inventory.

Whining. We have legitimate grievances that need to be aired from time to time. But becoming a complainer that no one wants around is all too easy. Pace yourself.

Blaming. It really doesn't matter who or what got you into this state. Inner peace requires working on our own stuff – not theirs.

Self-absorption. It does take a lot of inner vigilance to keep the ship running on course. But be sure to retain some interest in things outside yourself.

Shame. We've talked about this. Shame and guilt are big items in any psychological inventory. These things can really gum up the works. We may never get any further if we stop here.

Finally, watch out for *Fear*. It's normal to be afraid of insanity. A more pernicious fear, though, is the fear of living itself. To refuse opportunities for love or action or pleasure or achievement, because we 'might get sick' or we 'might not be up to it' is to shrink our lives to the size of a string bean. Make your reasonable best guess as to how you will handle it, and if it's not too awful, get out there.

There is something in all of us that would like to give up, go home, and hide under the covers. But there is also something we were meant to do, some talent we were meant to unfold, some goal that gives our life purpose. There is something that your spirit yearns for and is willing to do.

Fear is the great corrupter, not only of dreams but of honesty. It's also a sure sign we do not trust our Higher Power. Fear is the most corrosive emotion I know. I have a lot of it. Fear is what makes people collaborate with the enemy, and then beg and plead when they get executed anyway. Fear is not something to be indulged, it is to be fought. We can't always win. But people aren't sorry later for being brave, even if they lose. They're only sorry for being cowards.

Trust me, it hurts a lot less to go forward.

The Flip Side

Lastly, let me point out some good things that can be included in your inventory. Some people believe no inventory is complete until we add the positive things too.

I've mentioned some before, but they bear repeating. The PASC who manage to function in this complex world have many fine qualities, such as:

Endurance

Courage

Sensitivity

Insight

Depth

Hope

Humor

Compassion

Character

And remember, despite all this self-scrutiny, that we are far more than our flaws. We are not our disease; we are a person *with* a disease. Most of the time, we're doing our best. And God, however one pictures God, accepts us just that way.

Besides the reward of finding out about ourselves, we will have a great feeling of relief when we go forward to Step Five.

Outer Tips for Inner Peace

Strategy 4: Old Technology

Because of the possibility of unpredictable altered states, it is hard for many of the PASC to do significant paid work. Money is usually tight.

Yet the PASC, more than many, really need a computer. There are days and weeks when it may be our only contact and entertainment, our only way to function. But how can the PASC afford a computer? Lots of us can't.

However, the computer industry has a raging case of planned obsolescence, one of the curses of the modern world. Spend $3,000 on a computer system, and in six months it is outdated. The whole industry is rigged to make us buy over and over again.

If we're poor, of course, we can't do that (and it's kind of silly, anyway, don't you think?). *But other people will keep buying, to stay ahead of the curve.*

This is actually good news for the PASC. If you want life to be comfortable and not too prehistoric, cultivate 'old' technology. I don't mean 'ancient.' I mean the kind that just got downgraded because there is a New Thing for sale. Let your friends and family know that you are open to donations of working second-hand gadgets.

The modern world is bulging with cast-off computers. Nobody knows what to do with all of them – it is becoming a serious hard-waste problem. Ask your tech-savvy friends where to look for a good second-hand rig. Ask government employees or caseworkers or social workers how you can get one – qualify for a good one, say, on an educational program. Buddy up to your computer-owning friends and ask for their next hand-me-downs. The great thing about modern technology is that it is all pretty much made to work together – about the only serious exception is Mac versus PC, and even they are becoming more interchangeable. You can scrounge up an old monitor and keyboard and printer from three different species, and they can probably be made to work together.

If you actually want the Internet, and not just word processing, dial-up access is the cheapest way. Yes, the privileged complain that it is too slow – but if you are forced to listen to the demons in your head most days, what does it matter if a page takes 45 seconds to load instead of 25? All you need is a landline telephone of your own.

You should have one of these anyway. The one piece of technology no PASC person should ever be without is a way to IMMEDIATELY shout for help. Get one and keep it paid for – even if you must have someone else co-sign for it – even if all you ever dial is 911. I tend to recommend landlines over cell phones due to relative price and stability. If you can afford a cell phone, I'd still say keep a landline running. There are less likely to be network blank spots and run-out batteries just when you need them. Landlines also usually have discount programs for the disabled, which is not the case with cell phones.

So, get dial-up access to the Internet on your telephone. Access runs from inexpensive to free. You will have to ask your computer friends where the freebies are; my knowledge is sure to be outdated soon. There are also various companies that will offer you free service at certain hours of the day, or for a limited number of hours per month. Ask your hooked-up friends to search for one for you. If you get a laptop computer, you can always use the free networks in local coffeehouses. Once you have a computer hookup, you can shop for all the used hardware and peripherals and software your heart could desire on eBay or Craigslist, and many other places. There is never, never a shortage.

I know a very geeky poor man who keeps his home close to the cutting edge in this way: He saves $10 a week, that's all; and when the newest Mac product comes out, he buys the one that just went out of style (and dropped in price). These versions are still very competitive and will be good for years.

Apart from computers, what else can old tech do for you? Well, you may not be able to afford the latest iPhone, but you can have a fabulous collection of used CD's you picked up for pennies on the dollar, or a library of cassette tapes, or even a great vinyl collection if you have a phonograph – just keep the needle sharp. (No cheating will work there. You need new, first-rate needles.) And you don't have to *buy* all that music, either – consider the library. You might even get to borrow some of the very hottest top-ten items from their Teen collection. The library is better for people with older technology – many people donate cassette tapes, for instance. And as for traveling music – did you know that you actually get better sound quality from a Sony Walkman or mini CD player than from any MP3?

Then there is that 'dinosaur,' the VCR. Do you know how cheap those things are now? Have you ANY idea how many thousands of free video tapes have been donated to libraries in the last few years? You can amuse yourself with free classics for the rest of your life, or travel all around the world via free documentaries.

If all else fails, you can still sample all the music and news in your area with even the rattiest old radio.

And if you cannot find a free television, you're just not trying. I lived for 15 years without watching a TV, and people just kept donating them to me – at one time I had to give away FIVE just to keep the house boob-tube free.

So don't complain that you are the least and littlest Have-not in a neighborhood of Haves. Take advantage of it! Let them unload on you! You may never be on the cutting edge, but you can still have everything you need to be functional. Cultivate being content with substance rather than flash. Think of all that cash you are NOT throwing into the Great American Waste Machine. Take what you're offered with no false pride and a nice smile of thanks. People like to feel that they have benefited somebody with their 'junk.' Who knows? The next thing they throw out might be their iPad (or whatever the most recent gadget is), because they'd rather have the new version.

Just consider it your little freebie from the universe.

STEP FIVE

Admit Your Faults to Somebody

"Admitted to our Higher Power, ourselves, and another human being the exact nature of our wrongs."
- Adapted from the Twelve Steps of AA

STEP FIVE

To tell or not to tell? Or, in the case of the Fifth Step, whom to tell. That is the question.

Disclosure: it's a serious matter, in all parts of our lives. If you are able to function well enough to hide your disability, you probably do hide it - at least sometimes.

There is the matter of our own pride; but more importantly, there is the effect of stigma. How will it impact our lives if we tell? Will we be looked down upon, pitied? Will they be afraid of us, stop talking to us, whisper behind our backs? Will we lose our jobs, our lovers, our security clearance? Our driver's license? Our line of credit? Our good reputation? These are valid questions, not easily answered.

Shanna, who is 14, has had some mixed experiences with telling schoolmates.

> "I told a few friends, because they don't – a few of my friends have witnessed it. I had this friend for a long time whose name was Cindy. And I went through so much and she didn't understand that. I finally sat her down and talked to her; and then she got mad at me one day, for I don't know what – I was just – we were just talking one day and she was like, 'I gotta go,' and we were just talking, nothing bad, you know, just talking about our day. But: 'I gotta go.'

> "And then the next day I had all sorts of people calling me, telling me that she had called me a 'Bipolar' and then the 'b' word.

Like, spreading it around, telling everybody.
That was pretty bad.

"I still get called that every now and then.
But not that much.

"But [my boyfriend] – I told him pretty
much when we first started talking, because I
was going through so much at the time. So we
started talking, and I figured it would be best
to tell him.

"He didn't [know what it meant]. Most
people don't. He didn't really ask me
questions. He was scared to, because he didn't
know how I would react. We got talking one
day, and I said, 'Do you even know what
Bipolar is?' And he said, 'No, not really.' So I
was like, 'Why didn't you ask me? I had no
problem telling you. It doesn't hurt me, it kind
of helps me out.' He was like, 'Because I didn't
know if you'd think I was judging you, or
what.' He was very nice."

It's not uncommon that we not only have to disclose, we
then have to explain to other people what it is that we have just
disclosed! If they have heard the names of various special
chemistry conditions at all, they often have misconceptions.
Eddie generally opts for disclosure at work:

"When I work with people for a while, first I
slowly tell them – I hint around, then one day I
say, 'Look, you work with me every day, I'm
crippled through my destroyed leg, plus I have
a muscle disease'. They are more inclined to
believe me about the muscle disease, because
clearly, I wasn't lying about that [leg]. Then
after a while I say, 'You know, you've watched
me work and you see there's various

phenomena which I know you've got to be curious about. So the answer is – I'm nuts.' Then later I go, 'Here are the various meds that they use to, like, whatever.' People...the real-worlders, those who are *not obligated* to help, they're a little resistant at first: 'Oh, you're not crazy, you're not crippled.' But then I go, 'Well, here are the facts, that you can't refute,' and they're like, 'Oh, yeah, huh, that's wild. Wow. Huh. So, then, now what...blah blah blah?' and I go, 'Well, that blah blah blah.' And that's that...So long as it doesn't effect *them*, you don't really suffer from stigma."

Lisa handles it this way:

> "I only tell people that I know well and really trust that I'm Bipolar. I've heard too many people make fun of the condition to put myself out there for their ridicule...If someone behaves obnoxiously and irrationally, others joke about them being Bipolar...I know someone who openly told others she was Bipolar. Thereafter, if she so much as stated an opposing opinion in an argument she was dubbed a 'Bipolar bitch.' Society as a whole needs a prescription for hurtful labels."

Pablo, our Obsessive-Compulsive friend, keeps his experiences dead secret:

> "Through the years, my policy has been and still is to tell nobody. Unless I could discern that someone could have a real understanding, which is complicated to the point – unless someone has gone through similar things themselves, I feel it's impossible. So I don't tell anybody...

"Really, it's a great question. I'd like to sit in a room with many other people and see what their experiences were too. Because, people who are sort of going around with their everyday comings and goings, going to work and so forth, they don't give that a second thought.

"...Sometimes when you fill out an application form for something, it says, "Have you ever been diagnosed with' – I forget how the question goes. And I lie. I say, 'No, I haven't.' Who are they to know?

"...Because if you say to them, 'Oh, I was in Napa State Hospital for a year and 8 months,' they think, 'God – did you kill ten people?' "

Sally's experience is closer to my own: more disbelief than stigma.

"I tell people like I'm confessing. It's like we're intimate, if I tell you. 'I think you need to know in case you thought I was acting strange.' Most people don't know what [my diagnosis] means. If on the rare occasion that they should know, they say I'm too nice, I'm 'not that' at all. I haven't suffered from stigma, except my self-consciousness. Mostly, nothing has been bad about [my label], except the way I penalize myself with what the label means according to psychology."

Sally has just pinpointed another reaction we sometimes get. People who like us, and are convinced that special chemistry is 'bad,' simply will deny that we have it. Somehow they think this is a kindness. But what they are doing is denying us the support we need.

Shanna has such a dynamic with her own father.

"I know a lot of people who have been through a lot worse...But it helped to have a supportive mom. My dad would be supportive if he understood. But he doesn't understand, so he can't be supportive.

"...We called him when we found out I was Bipolar for real, you know, the actual diagnosis, and then he came home and he just told me that it was OK. 'It's OK, you're really mild Bipolar, if you are at all.' That's what he told me. He said, 'You're very, very mild Bipolar, you're not crazy,' is what he told me.

"Hey, I'm not 'crazy' even if I'm extremely Bipolar! Because it's not something you can help.

"...Momma pretty much had to make Daddy let me go [get help].

"My dad, though, he's never gone to a mental health clinic or anything, because I don't let him. He doesn't know about any of that stuff. He knows that I was pretty much psychotic, for a while? But he thinks – every time Momma talks to him about it, he says that I just have a temper.

"He is in denial. Daddy has taken psychology because he's a warden and everything, he has to deal with psychotic inmates. But when it comes to his own daughter, I'm pretty sure he doesn't want to admit it.

"So I've had to tell him – I went on a really bad phase one time, and I told him that I needed to go to the hospital. And Momma understood. She said, 'Okay, I'll go talk to your Daddy.' Daddy refused to take me.

"I was bad. I was extremely bad that night. And I told Momma, if I didn't go to the hospital, something extremely bad was going to happen. I pretty much was planning really bad stuff that night. Even though I was on my medicine, I was planning evil stuff. It was a breakdown."

Sometimes we can find ourselves in the odd position of having to convince our friends and intimates that we really do have a condition, just to get the support we require.

Outside of our intimate circle, however, often the easiest thing to do is try to 'pass' for normal, much like light-skinned Africans sometimes used to 'pass' for white to survive in the early twentieth century. We think it will save us trouble.

But not telling can be just as bad. We are then required to live a lie, make up excuses, and somehow try to function at a 'normal' level even though it exhausts us and doesn't really work. Author Joanne Greenberg, writing from the perspective of a Schizophrenic just released and learning to live in the 'normal' world, describes it this way:

All Deborah heard were her gasps of exhaustion as she climbed an Everest that was to everyone else an easy and level plain...Why had she been so pitifully proud? She had given all her strength, all her struggle, all her will to succeed...Now it was over and what had it been, after all, but what everyone else did without half trying?...It had taken all her capacities, every drop of her will, to come as far as

*they had come laughing and easy...the world offered
its immense beauty, but she would burn away all
her strength just staying alive.*

--*Joanne Greenberg, I Never Promised You a Rose Garden*

Then there is the moral problem involved in such a lie.
What about the 'rigorous honesty' so often advised in the
Twelve-Step 'Big Book'? Also there is a question of social
responsibility. If we 'fake normal,' aren't we just supporting the
stigma and making it harder for the generations that follow?

Theoretically, this is not a problem in the Twelve-Step
fellowship. This is the place where everyone is welcome,
regardless of their past, right? Is special chemistry less
acceptable than shooting up? Stealing to support a habit? Going
to jail? Beating your kids during a drunken binge? Where do we
draw the line?

Perhaps it is not so much a question of 'better' or 'worse.'
The operative word here is 'different.' OK, maybe we *are*
different. Maybe you are the only one in the room with your
particular problems and symptoms; although I doubt it.
Virtually every time I come clean about this at a Twelve-Step
meeting, at least one person thanks me afterwards and reveals a
psychiatric condition of their own – or if not theirs, a family
member's.

However, let's suppose you are the only one in your
meeting or your area. Do you disclose? Or do you not?

It's a personal decision. Don't allow it to interfere with
your progress, one way or another. That's the bottom line. Our
sanity is always the top priority. Isolation and loneliness are
part of the old, sick pattern. One of the ways we get and keep
recovery is by breaking this pattern wherever we can. This does
not mean we must bring up our special chemistry at every
single meeting. But if it's relevant, if it's affecting our spiritual
life today, then we can feel free to mention it as part of the
sharing process.

Luckily, when it comes to the Fifth Step, there is no
dilemma. We *must* admit everything, to at least one person, and

to whatever Power we acknowledge. Keeping our weakness to ourselves is not an option.

Disclosure and Dating

My experience is that somewhere in our lives we need to disclose. People need other people. People need to be understood. People need to be seen and accepted for exactly what they are. Isolation is not only painful, it is prejudicial to our growth. And in our case it can even be lethal. Suicide is a chronic issue for some of us. Self-imposed death is the ultimate in isolation: it is not likely to happen to a person who feels sufficiently accepted and understood.

Nowhere in life is this more obvious than in the sexual realm. Again and again, men who were PASC told me that they found they were rejected by women because of their special chemistry – or more commonly, for the poverty caused by special chemistry.

I asked each of my interview subjects what the worst thing was that they had experienced as a result of mental illness. Pablo originally said his medical overdose – a story we'll get to – was the worst. Later he changed his answer:

> "True, being overdosed was a harrowing experience; but that came to an end. What has been most painful for me is the impossibility of securing a meaningful and loving relationship...I began to understand that no woman would want to deal with me and the Obsessive-Compulsive behavior. Oh, I might have found such a person at length, but that might have taken 50 years and there was not the luxury of that much time."

One point I would like to make here, though, is that Pablo never in his life was medically treated for Obsessive-Compulsive Disorder. He had a horrendous early experience with a hospital (see Step 8) and never trusted the medical establishment again. I think it likely that if he had allowed himself to receive proper treatment, it would have been possible for him to find a partner. But we'll never know.

Eddie describes his dating difficulties in this tongue-in-cheek way:

> "One other area. Dating. But that's not so much stigma. The girls are not really...I mean, [it's] just to assuage their guilt. If you weren't answering a personals ad, like if you could go around it, find out who they are, and then approach them and make it look like an accident, and just say, 'Hey, here's a weird story for you; there's this mentally ill guy who has to be on medication,' they'd just be like, 'Oh. Well, glad he's getting help.' Right?

> "But then they have to fake like they're sickened by it when they enter the official dating realm. Because if they don't make you morally culpable in that realm – if in fact you are an innocent guy who's perfectly worthy – then the question is why are they being so greedy? Which is a question not to ask in our culture. So they have to say, they have to announce in their ads, 'All people with the following problems are really unethical, shameful *losers*, and so why would I debase myself that way?' But that's *only* in that arena.

> "But if you end-ran it, if you said, 'This person won't be dating you, this person won't be related to you, so you wouldn't have an obligation that way...how do you feel about a guy who went kind of nuts and had to be on medication and now he seems kind of normal?' They'd say, 'Right on.' Or whatever.

"So in dating specifically, and not in the whole of those women's lives, but when they must enter the monetary and logistical thing... they kind of have to be ruthless.

"...If you had a sufficient amount of money it wouldn't matter...for instance, if you're wealthy – and I've often said this – and you, say, 'Yeah, I'm sorry that I can only date you twice a week because I'm so claustrophobic. To make up for it, all the hurt feelings you have, why don't I buy you a trip to Palm Springs for a week, and just pay your salary that you'll be missing.' There's a lot of forgiveness there. [laughter] Yeah, you know, I'm so sorry that I'm too Depressed to have sex. Let's get you a new car and hire a fulltime masseuse to come every day, to give you physical attention.' There's just a *lot* of forgiveness there!

"I've tested this. I've written back and said, 'You know how you didn't want anyone with psychological or physical problems? I do, I have all those problems, and it's weird of a guy who's a multimillionaire like I am to have all those problems. But I'm hoping that you'll see your way around that and start dating me so I could see if my three-month trip to Tuscany is something you could do with me.' They'll get over it."

Some people solve this problem by only dating other special chemistry people. But this can be hazardous – our partners may not be available to help us at critical times because they are having symptoms of their own. And it is not a good idea to start seeing ourselves as only able to attract people with psychological problems.

Jessica, the post-graduate student, has gotten a mixed bag of responses from friends and coworkers in regard to her multiple conditions:

> "Sometimes they'll walk on eggshells around me. Sometimes they don't really say anything, but I can tell maybe they're uncomfortable. Sometimes they'll tell me I need to get off all my psych medications right away because they're making me crazier. I've had people that I was working for do that...one of them, she had me so freaked out ...she was, like, making me feel like she couldn't let me work for her any more...I ended up having a Panic Attack...by the end of the week I was in the emergency room."

She has nevertheless been in her current live-in relationship for ten years. Even among perfectly healthy people, that's an accomplishment.

What I have found works best is to stick with people of character – people who have some education about psychological matters, perhaps; or who have some experience with compassion; or who are for whatever reason willing to be flexible. These are usually high-quality people. The best strategy is to tell them about your special chemistry after they have some experience of how your character works *outside* the disease.

I told my now-husband after we had been having serious long talks over the telephone for more than two months. We had even discussed our views on abnormal psychology. I felt he knew me fairly well, and had a balanced view of the PASC. I could certainly have waited longer, but it came up in conversation on our second in-person date, and I decided to use the natural opening.

After I explained, I gave him a bright smile and said, "I will understand completely if you decide to run for the hills!" I still don't know why he didn't, but that was his choice. I was ready to let him go if he felt he couldn't face it.

This was in the context of a deepening attachment, where we both knew the possible stakes were marriage. It was a moral responsibility to tell him sooner or later. I already knew he was a caring man who had nursed a previous wife through a number of illnesses. I knew he was not afraid of imperfection.

If all you want is a one-night stand, of course, it need never come up.

It is important to have a core group of supporters, and often this does mean people with similar problems. It's a relief, sometimes, to 'talk shop': swap stories of the most bizarre things we've done, laugh about them. Gossip and complain about doctors and the failures of the mental health system; even trade morbid stories about the various methods of suicide, and how close we've come. Why not? Stuntmen exchange tales of near-disasters, too, and nobody finds that strange or threatening. We feel a sense of safety and relief when we know we're not the only ones. I will never forget the tale of a girlfriend who could not figure out the safety on her husband's gun. She was so determined to kill herself that she went to the library to look it up! They figured out what she was doing and had her taken to the hospital.

I really recommend that you try not to make a nuisance of yourself by discussing your mental condition with normies too often, though. There are some basic facts and news reports your intimates need, true – but just think of how tiresome it is when people go on and on about their personal health. There's such a thing as etiquette. There's such a thing as saving their sympathy for times when you really need it.

But we need not limit ourselves to fellow-sufferers entirely. It's important to keep relating to the mainstream. If we get too exclusive, we may start believing that only 'damaged' people can love us or relate to us — and that would be a tragic mistake.

So, in terms of choosing somebody to whom to read your Fifth Step, be picky but don't go overboard. If we can find a dual-diagnosis person to read to, this is ideal. If we have been admitting our illness at meetings, we probably know who they are. Or we can quietly ask around. Maybe we have a strong bond with our sponsor[1], or a particular person just gives us a good, warm, accepted feeling.

If we are PASC, even without a substance abuse problem, we probably already have a core of people who know about us.

You might also consider doing Fifth-Step disclosure with your therapist. I'd recommend this at least as an aid to Fifth-Step work. Probably there are as many ways to use therapy as there are people using it. But ultimately, therapy is about finding your personal truth. So therapy can be an excellent place to read your inventory. It is safe, it is private, and if you're doing your part, it's as rigorously honest as you're ever likely to get. At the very least, if you're stuck on these Steps, you can think over your last few therapy sessions and get a clue as to where you hurt, where you most need change and healing.

If you approach your Fifth Step with someone unfamiliar with your special chemistry, be prepared to give a thumbnail sketch to bring that person up to speed. It needn't be a lecture. Just a brief summary of what you've got and how it affects you. Don't get drawn into a long-winded discussion of various aspects, including medications, side effects, and number and length of hospitalizations. It's probably not wise to finish a Fifth Step with anybody who seems morbidly fascinated. All we need is for someone to accept this as an important factor in our lives (like knowing a diabetic has to watch their blood sugar).

A side note about therapists and doctors: you may occasionally find a doctor (not a top one) who wants you to discuss "what it feels like" every time you come in. Unless they are looking for clues to prevention, this is inappropriate. Tell them firmly that you can't describe it and that this is not helpful to you. If they keep poking at it, find another doctor. They have missed the point, and are off on some trip of their own. I have encountered this twice, and never got much good out of either of those professionals.

---

[1] A 'sponsor' is a mentor within the Twelve Step program whom you request to help you along the way. In program, you may ask anyone, but they can choose whom to accept. We all need mentors, and if you can find someone more experienced in your condition than you are, this is tremendously helpful.

We can also look among the organizations dedicated to helping PASC people. Some of these are groups of fellow sufferers; some are families and caretakers who want to understand. These are valid, safe places to be honest. I will list some resources to start off with at the end of this book.

As for the original question of whether to disclose your condition to those around you, I have no easy answers. My personal system is to tell on a need-to-know basis. Will my illness affect my tenancy? If not, I don't have to tell my landlord. Will it affect my ability to perform at work? If not, it's not my boss's business. Also, I use my intuition and common sense as to who can handle this information in an adult, non-stigmatic manner.

Of course, any serious boyfriend/girlfriend, all really close friends, and medical workers need to know the truth. And I never lie about it if someone asks me point-blank. But if I had epilepsy, or a heart condition − or poison ivy, for god's sake − would I feel compelled to say this to someone interviewing me for a new job? No. Why would they need to know that? And it's the same with our choice to disclose. It's a medical condition − no more or less − and we have a right to decide who knows about it. Otherwise, it's just not relevant.

I tend to tell anyone who I feel can deal with the information. I do think it's important for people to see for themselves that the PASC are not necessarily scary or dangerous. I like to think that in some future time, someone will profit because I helped dispel the myth today. (It may be just a delusion, but it helps me sleep at night.)

I gave long thought to whether I'd use my own name for this book. In the end, I felt that helping to end stigma was more important than protecting myself.

On the whole, I'd say honesty is still the best policy...if your audience can handle it.

As Shelley, the special education teacher, told me,

"I think it's kinda cool. Because one of those questions you have there [in your interview] is, What would you tell the world,

you know, if you could, about having mental
illness? If you could give one piece of advice to
people that have it? It would be to share with
other people! That it ain't so bad! It's OK to be
'off' – you know, whatever that means…It's a
chemical imbalance! It's something that a lot of
people have. It's very, very common. And not
to hide it from people. PLEASE don't hide it
from people!"

There's a difference between being open and being a
pest, though. The day I wrote this, I was a little Manick-y, a little
confused, and I had to drive down to the supermarket anyway.
I was so off balance that I started to walk off without paying.
When the checker called me back, I apologized and said, "I'm
out of it today. I keep making mistakes."
        The checker said casually, "Got too much on your
mind?"
        And I blurted out, "I have a mental condition."
        She looked very taken aback, and replied, "Oh, I didn't
mean to get personal."
        I responded, "It's nothing much. I'm just waiting for a
pill to kick in," and her face relaxed once more.
        I'm not saying she was actually frightened, but it was
too much information, and it was inappropriate.
        It was a national holiday, and there she was, working. So
I said, "Be sure to do something nice for yourself this evening,"
and left her smiling. I hope that made up for her moment's
discomfort.
        But I should know better. I've been doing this for, what,
30 years?
        There are times when we may feel people need
educating, or we may have principles about bringing something
out in the open. But I felt I had crossed the comfort line when
there was no need. You'll have to determine your own
boundaries between what is self-respectful and what is just
hiding out.
        And like me, you'll make mistakes. Doesn't everybody?

Outer Tips to Inner Peace

Strategy 5: Try The Library

Most of the PASC are unable to work full time. And yet, we are not so sick we can just lie down and take pills all day. That often leaves a dilemma of too much leisure time and too little money.

The biggest bang for your buck is almost always the local library. Most people have no idea of all that's available there. I do know, because I worked at one for 12 years. The library is the best free entertainment in town.

For one thing, it's a quiet, safe place to go where no one will bother you. Librarians tend to be tolerant people and believe in their duty to *all* members of the public. Even if you are talking to yourself or haven't combed your hair this week, if you leave the other patrons in the library alone, the librarians will probably let you be. You don't need a library card to read the magazines and newspapers on site. A major library carries more titles and subjects than you can even imagine – you will probably never waste cash on a subscription again!

Getting a card is usually easy and free. You show some kind of ID and proof of your address. This can be as simple as an envelope from your electric bill. They may even give you a postcard to send to yourself, if you don't have other proof of where you live.

Of course there are books that can teach you anything you want – including plenty about your special chemistry, how to navigate the government agencies, and your legal rights. But there is so much more! There are phone books from dozens of places. There is a reverse directory where you can look up a phone number and get the name or address. There is a reference librarian to help you find things – he or she is the original search engine, and is amazingly happy to use his or her skills for you. Beyond that, there are library databases that will sort a subject out for you better than 10 hours of googling.

But suppose you're just not into books? There is still plenty there for you.

If your condition makes it hard to read, there are often records, tapes, CDs, videos and DVDs to check out – who needs Netflix? – and even music scores. There may be a branch which loans out tools. The art and photography volumes can take you through the greatest museums in the world. There are maps to everywhere. There are language tapes to learn with. There are atlases and pamphlets on local government services. There are art and craft exhibits. There are extra rooms where seminars and lectures and club meetings take place – everything from poetry readings to free tax help and more.

Should you happen to have children, there are often programs for them, or a Story Hour, or under-the-desk items such as crayons and scissors and colored paper for children to use if you ask nicely. The library is NOT a free babysitter – but it can be a better alternative to television or video games, at least for an hour or two.

And of course, there are computers. This might be the greatest boon to the financially challenged. You can get a free email account (such as hotmail) and check your mailbox. Using the computer usually requires signing up in advance, so be sure to call or ask ahead of time. You can surf and search to your heart's content in the hour or half-hour given to you – just come in with a list of exactly what to look for, lest you get sidetracked and waste your limited time. You can apply for things, look for apartments, and make printouts (possibly for a small fee like 5 cents a page). You can watch videos, read the New York Times, and all the things that people love to do on the World Wide Web, and it won't cost you a penny. They may even give computer lessons in those seminar rooms I mentioned.

You can sometimes get extra time on the computers as a disabled person, if you have trouble concentrating or understanding. It's worth at least applying for the privilege. You may also be able to get other privileges such as extended check-out periods. Libraries are careful to make resources open to everybody.

Be scrupulous about returning items on time and in good condition. If you do lose something for a long time, you won't be charged the earth for it; there is usually a maximum amount, which won't be more than the item is worth. And once every few years, or decades, the library might even stage an 'amnesty period' where anyone can return old items for free and get their record wiped clean. I just hope you'll never need that!

Apart from anything else, the library is a safe, clean, quiet place to hang out – maybe the only one in your neighborhood, if your living quarters are bottom of the barrel. It may also be a better place to meet with people than in your room, if your room is small or depressing.

Librarians are usually sincere souls who believe devoutly in the dignity and rights of everyone. Get to know them, and they will repay you with attention and great service.

This is absolutely your safest place to spend time, if you can't stand the inside of your head any longer.

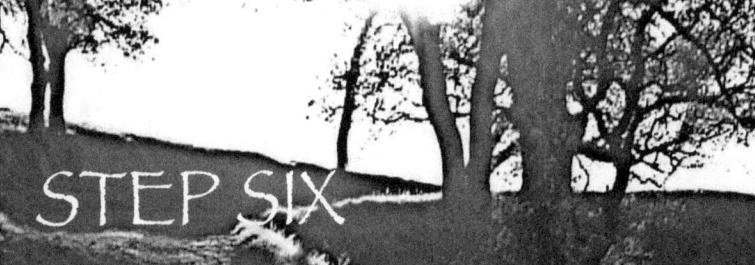

STEP SIX

Get Ready to Improve

"Became entirely ready to have
our Higher Power remove all
these defects of character".

STEP SEVEN

Get Help Improving

"Humbly asked our
Higher Power
to remove our
shortcomings".

- Both adapted from the Twelve Steps of AA

Steps Six and Seven

Human nature is a contrary thing. On the one hand, we yearn to be perfect (usually using some TV hero as a model). On the other hand, we believe deep down that we are right about most things, and we really don't want anybody picking around in our conscience. That includes God.

This is especially true when some piece of oneself was created as a defense. Parents aren't perfect, adolescents are cruel, and we all end up with some painful bumps and dents built into our psyches. To guard against living through such pain again, we naturally build defenses. The problem is, 20 years down the road they are obsolete, and may even become obstacles to living the life we now want.

There are also our built-in oddities, which need not grow into problems but so often do. Some folks just seem to have been born angry or impatient. Some people have been afraid of everything from the cradle (and some seem to have been naturally equipped with charm and the ability to take things in stride – but we won't talk about those weirdos). Maybe a tendency toward leadership turns into pushiness. Or an ability to endure becomes plain mule stubbornness. We don't necessarily want to remove these traits. We think it would be enough just to tone them down.

And besides, these things feel familiar and safe. They're part of our very identity. Do we really want to change? Would we know the person that was left?

The fact is change has already caught up with you. If our disease were lifted completely tomorrow morning, we would not return to exactly who we were when mental illness split our lives open. We have learned things about being on the marginal side of society. About pain. About horrendous loss of control. Possibly we lost a lot of friends, and we won't feel the same about them, either. Possibly we became deadly poor, and found out more about the insurance industry and its limits than we ever wanted to know. Certainly, we would never hear about cuts to mental health services with indifference again. We would feel new sympathy and new understanding. We would never take a sane, clear mind for granted any more.

And since you have NOT been miraculously cured, brace yourself. You are only going to encounter further shifts as you go on.

No matter how much lip service we pay to the idea, most of us really don't want change. We are as comfortable in our faults as in a stretchy old armchair just right for our bottoms. We say, 'Aw, who wants to be perfect, anyway?' We are even willing to get the same old bad results, as long as we don't have to do anything very new or different. (If you doubt this, look at the eerily similar messes that we make over and over with the same kind of love partner!) Part of it is just habit. Part of it is the sneaky but misguided belief that we are right. Part of it is just plain old fear of the unknown, the best reason of all. We get into self-change mostly by accident.

It's much like an addiction. We do things the same old way no matter how much it hurts until one day it hurts *too much*. We turn to change as a last option. We turn to it with a secret agenda. We are going to *control* the way we change. We are only going to change an inch or so, maybe just temporarily, and then stop.

People often go into therapy in this mood. They really want the therapist to come up with a magic formula, and if she can't, she can at least not fiddle with our innards. Not much, anyway. We only want such and such a problem solved. It seems easy. Just tell me what to say to shift the problem off my shoulders. It shouldn't hurt. Well, only a little. Certainly God should have nothing to do with it.

The Sixth and Seventh Steps don't let us hide in ways like these. Someone else, the One who sees everything, will decide when and where and how our transitions will happen. Therefore, it will probably hit from a surprising direction.

It requires hope beyond the norm. It takes imagination. But I also think it is a matter of squaring up to reality. Life does not generally give us a choice about what lessons we are going to be called on to learn.

Sally finds that the whole ordeal has strengthened her faith:

> "I believe everything is in divine order and divine timing. I believe I have a good life. I believe everything happens for a reason. I believe I can serve God through the trials I have been through. Because of my story, I have come to nestle in the arms of God in a real way much faster than I would have if I had not been through hard times.
>
> "...I have become more of a lady. I have become more proper. It has shaped me because I overcompensate for my character. I'm good at a lot of things because of this flawed feeling. I can't say this is a bad thing."

On the news and in movies and books, we are constantly exposed to the worst things that humans can do. Sometimes it seems there is no bottom to it. But what about the *best* that humankind can do? Have you ever, for instance, tried to envision a world with no war and no hunger? It's kind of mind-boggling. There are souls who give their entire lives trying to build such a world. But let's bring it to the personal level. Try to imagine: what would you be like if every anger and error and fear were peeled right off you like the skin of a peach? Who would you be if you were perfectly OK? What are the UPPER limits of humankind's behavior? Have we ever tried to find out? Wouldn't it be worth a little pain and uncertainty to get there?

Lisa speculates about it:

> "But I often wonder what I would have been like if I'd possessed a more normal

childhood and an existence free of mental disorders. Would I be a more peaceful, happy person, or would I be more selfish and uncaring, or any other number of trait combinations? Of course there is no way to know, but I'm still curious."

Let me tell you a little story about myself. My mental illness flowered at the same time as puberty hit me. I did not find out that there was a reason for the way I acted until I was 26 years old. At that point, I was already a divorced alcoholic who stood up her friends, kept them waiting for no reason, yelled at them, and slept with their best buddies, among other things. So I had very few friends. My job was also in jeopardy, though I didn't know it. I began to take lithium and gained some control over my actions. I was deeply ashamed of the unkind parts of my life. But what I didn't realize was that I was still not free of symptoms. I still verbally abused people close to me and could not stick to any long-term plans. I still became hysterical over small stresses. I didn't know this was abnormal, however, because since childhood, I had never experienced anything else.

Most people become PASC in their early adult years. They have an idea of who they are before all the changes set in. Not me. I had never even been a normal teenager. I had no idea who I was, underneath my symptoms.

The fact is, we are all in that same boat when it comes to character flaws. We don't really know, and probably can't imagine, what we would be like without our human defects. My guess is that it would be something beautiful, something the world could certainly use. Yet we can't do it alone. We must have a Higher Power's help, asking It to help us remove our flaws as It sees fit. We give it our best shot; then we wait. Wait to see how the Universe will react. It will.

If you want to know the end of my story, I am happy to tell you that the best drug therapy for me was discovered when I was 34. Almost overnight, I became a different person. A person I could like. A person other people could live with. A person who could make up her mind, make plans, and most of the time stick to them. *A person I didn't have to be ashamed of.* It was very much a miracle, one for which I am grateful every day.

I'm not saying that you should expect an instant miracle. But leave room for one to happen. Just in case.

Very seldom does it happen, however, that faults are simply taken from us wholesale. Remember that this is an interactive universe. It will probably confront us with whatever fault we decide we want to work on. If we decide we need to be more patient, for instance, we will instantly be put at the end of a very long line!

Or maybe we want to start taking things less personally. This is a good one for most of the PASC. We tend to be self-absorbed in our Depression, Compulsion, Paranoia, Anxiety, or Manic phases. We tend to take every remark or happening as if it were intended just for us. So let's say we decide to work on detachment.

What will happen is that the universe will throw these situations in our way, repeatedly. Somebody says something to us that can be interpreted two ways, one of them insulting. Do we get upset, offended? Or do we back off and consider, "Maybe so-and-so is just irritated in general. Maybe he is getting an ulcer, or a divorce." Do we get all worked up, or let it slide off us like water off a duck's back? If we can't detach this time, don't worry – it will surely come up again, and again. I promise, there's plenty of practice, once you have picked a characteristic to work with.

And suppose someone says something that is genuinely critical of us? It still behooves us to detach. For one thing, unless that person is important to us, who cares what they think? That's their reality – that's how they see it – fine, we don't have to agree. If the speaker is our boss or a loved one, it is still smart to detach. Detachment works a lot better than obsessing over the remark, or going off like fireworks.

Once we feel we've got the hang of it, we will be tested. The truism goes that the universe tests us three times, just to see if we've really got the point. So don't be surprised if it comes up a few more times, even when you think you've moved on.

And we will move on. This is a lifelong process. It's called spiritual evolution, and it's not really optional – unless we are fully committed to being jerks for life.

Outer Tips for Inner Peace

Strategy 6: Entertainment

If your mental state is fragile, you might want to watch what kind of entertainment you pour into your head. I'm not the kind of prude who says no sex, violence, or swearing. But there is a big difference between seeing a fast car chase or a building blowing up, and watching somebody's fingers cut off, one by one, right in your face. Depressed people don't need to see the rotting flesh slip off a zombie's face. Paranoid people shouldn't search for movies about corrupt governments or conspiracies that crush the poor and the weak. If Anxiety is your problem, you shouldn't see something that will give you nightmares.

Just consider how you're going to feel when you get home. Are you going to be frightened? Terminally sad? Despairing at the state of the world? Not everything has to have a happy ending; just be aware of possible after-effects. You can usually tell from the movie previews or from the dust jackets of books and videos or DVDs. A lot of times, the things that are 'critically acclaimed' are complete downers. Sometimes you need something trivial and light. There's a lot to be said for Public Television, too. And nothing is stopping you from turning off the news if it's horrifying.

It is hard enough to live with what's already in your head. Don't put lots more ugly images there. You might bump into them at 3 a.m. some morning.

Strategy 7: Emotional Input

You might also consider the conversational ambience around you. I don't mean you should make Positive Thinking your religion. Survival for the PASC requires realism. But if talking to certain people always seems to leave you feeling worse, maybe you should spend less time with them. If a conversation seems centered on the more upsetting things in the world, try to change the subject. If they're stuck on scary, drift off in some other direction.

I had a friend who was going through a desperate Depression. I offered myself as a sounding board, not knowing how critical his condition would get. Soon I was getting two or three letters a day telling me how horrible and without hope his life was, and how much he wanted to die. By the time I finished reading these letters, *my* day was ruined. And since I wasn't even there in person looking sympathetic, I wasn't doing him much good.

There was more. Bit by bit, because of my sympathy, he leaned on me harder for favors and care. I suddenly realized one day that I had promised to take his cat if he died, be executor of his considerable estate (he sent me pages and pages of new handwritten instructions every week), find him a new home in case he survived – and it had to be a really nice one for a dirt-cheap price – and on and on. One day I got a call from his bank informing me that he wished to give me financial control over all the money he had left in the world. I found myself calling his therapist and having long conversations with her about such things as how to get him to give up his guns.

That's when I had to pull the plug. I realized then that in his despair, he wanted to give complete control of his life to someone else.

I could understand that. *But I was not up for the job.* I was PASC too, and I had PASC problems of my own, which were being made worse by trying to rescue him. I had to tell him I was only going to be executor, nothing else. He was very angry at me, and though I didn't blame him, I could not afford to change my decision. It was hard enough running my own PASC life. I could not run his, too.

I'm afraid that man died. Yes, by his own hand. There were other people receiving multiple letters, and being asked for unmanageable amounts of support; other people going nuts trying to raise him out of his Depression, and *none* of us could save him. What he really needed was a hospital, and he wouldn't go.

We have to think about what we are taking on. No matter how much compassion we may feel, there are limits to how much we can actually do for someone. We may perfectly understand how they feel, but be unable to manage because of our own limitations. We are simply not up to the task. You do have the right to say, "I am not a professional, and I can't handle this." It's OK to say, "I understand, but I can't fix this."

This may sound harsh. But tell me, who else is going to protect us, if we don't? We are grown up. It's not anybody else's job, any more. It is our moral imperative, as thinking, choosing people of free will, to take care of ourselves. And it is that other person's responsibility to care for his or her own self. It is NOT our responsibility to take care of them, even though we might desperately wish we could. Few of us really have the resources to save someone else's mind, heart, or body.

I am not saying we should not care for each other. I am saying that you and I are PASC, we have certain serious limitations, and we cannot afford to pull someone else from the edge of the abyss *if they are going to pull us over with them*. If we cannot help, we must let go. We must leave the rescue work to those who are trained for it.

If someone needs THAT much of a buffer from reality, if someone needs to be watched over night and day, they should be in the hospital (as my poor friend should have been).

Have compassion, but don't insist on rescuing everybody else. You must retain enough energy to save yourself! It's *your* job.

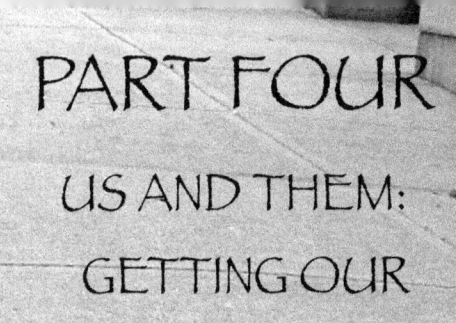

PART FOUR

US AND THEM: GETTING OUR STORIES STRAIGHT

"To say that nobody cared about people with psychiatric problems... was to put it kindly. What people really wanted, he suspected, was for the neurobiologically ill simply to vanish. Get out of sight. Go away. Die. They were just too unpleasant. They raised too many questions..."
— <u>Straw Girl</u>

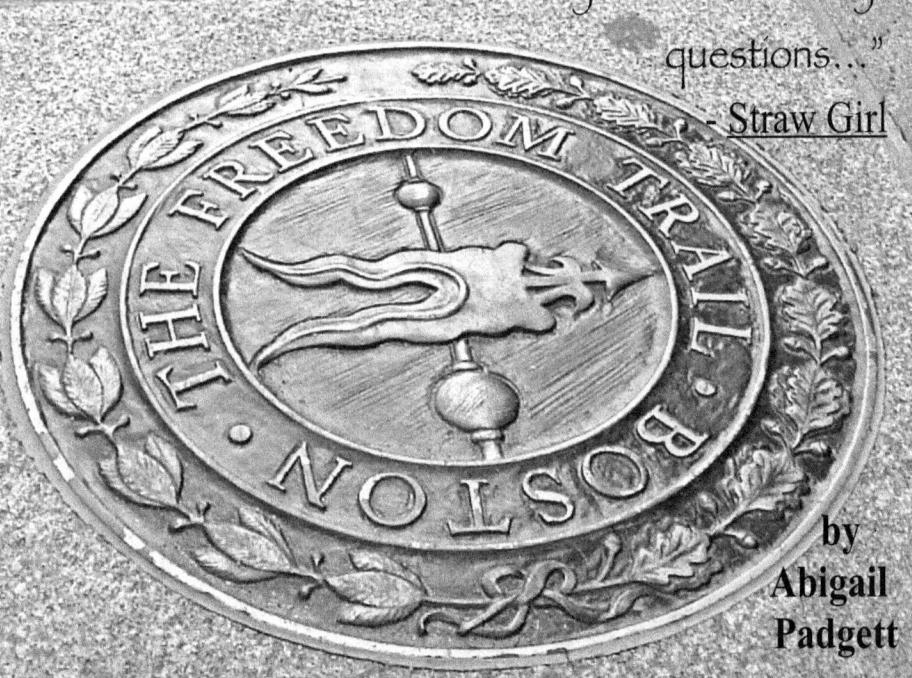

by
Abigail
Padgett

STEP EIGHT

Get Ready to Face the Damage You've Done

"Made a list of all persons we had harmed
and became willing to make amends to them all."

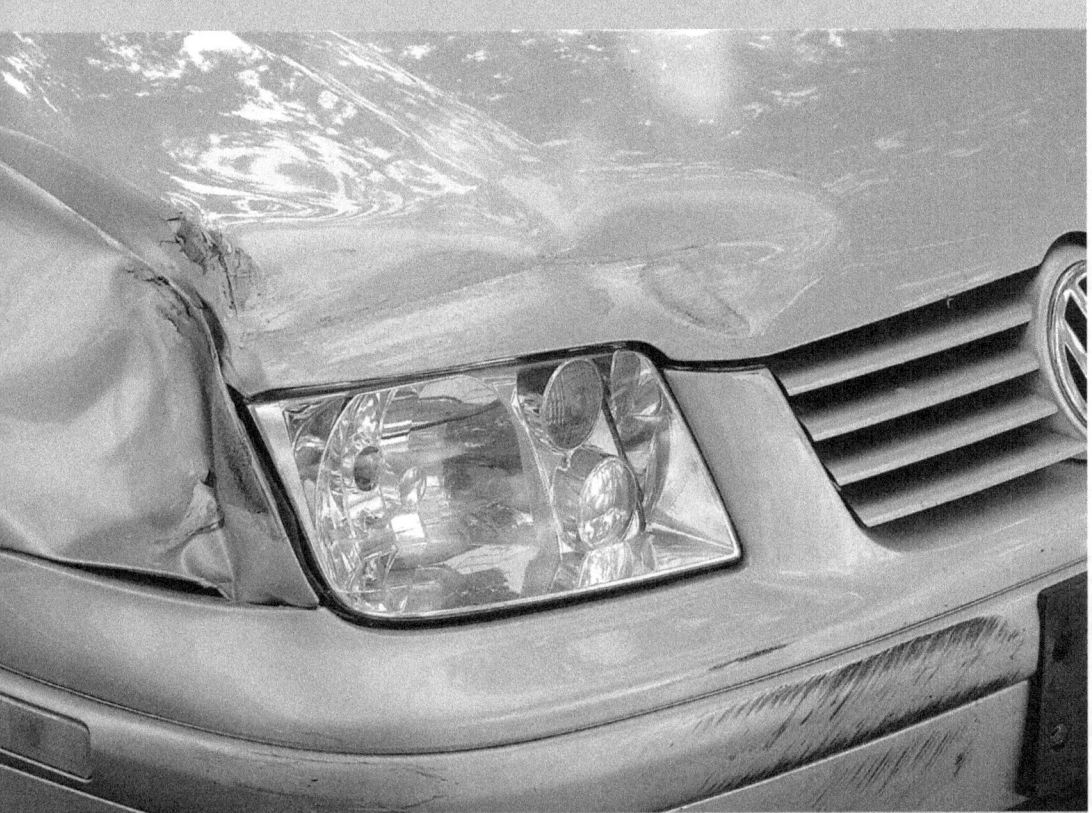

STEP NINE:

Atone for Damages

"Made amends to these persons wherever possible
except where it might harm them or others."
-Both adapted from the Twelve Steps of AA

Steps Eight and Nine

You may remember, back in Step Four, that I advised you to make a list of your worst and most harmful episodes, and put it aside for later. This is later. Time to deal with the harm we've done to other people.

But, wait, says someone in the back row. What about the harm they've done to us?

I was afraid you'd bring that up.

I have tried, throughout this book, to maintain a positive note and a tone of optimism. But the way the general public treats the mentally ill is not pretty.

Before you can ask forgiveness from those you've harmed, you must deal with the wounds that some of those very same people have dealt to you. Shelley remembers a lot of bad press:

> "I have been invited to parties, say, with a certain group of people, in past years – you know, over the years, I'm talking decades here – a group of people I would know and then the word would get out, 'Shelley's Manic Depressive.' And, 'Oh, my God.' One of the women – it was always a woman. Always a woman saying, 'no more of her.' Always a woman saying, 'she sucks, she's bad news, she's going to destroy our kitchen, there's going to be fruit flying everywhere, glasses breaking.'"

So, little as I like it, it's time for a bit of mud-slinging.

What They've Done To Us

Nelson from the United Kingdom is quite clear about what special chemistry has done to his life. "I have lost my job, my ability to support my family, and the respect of my wife." Isn't this exactly the scenario that everyone fears?

One of the scarier tales I have heard comes from our Obsessive-Compulsive friend Pablo. Pablo experienced a Depression in his twenties which was somehow misdiagnosed as Schizophrenia, and he nearly died of the treatment. I tell his story here at length.

Receiving an unexpected inheritance through his wife, Pablo decided to buy them a house. It was his first time, and it turned out to be a bad move in a number of ways.

The neighborhood, the distance from work, the change in finances, and the condition of the house itself were all negatives. Pablo is also subject to Clinical Depression, and he had his first experience with it then.

> "My first thought was, I'd made an error. I'd made a catastrophic error. And there was no way to back out. That was the way my thinking went...And so I just went down, down, down, down, *down*, till I got so Depressed, I couldn't go to work. I had the inability to deal – most people can – you know, you make a mistake...deal with it successfully! What happened was, the Depression, it simply didn't lift. Because my thought was there was no way out. And when you start thinking [like that] – so, for the only time in my life, I attempted suicide.

> "It was really a very serious test run. It wasn't a – [I] feel sort of embarrassed about it after all these years! It was purposeful in its intent. I jumped in the bathtub and filled it up with water, I plugged in an electric heater, and

I dumped it into the bathtub with me. What happened was, the heater shorted out!

"Obviously things were so serious; that's when, rightly so, my wife said, 'We can't go on with this, you know,' and I said, 'Yeah.' My folks made arrangements then – I don't know how they did it – to have me admitted to [a local high-profile facility]. So that's where things went bad to worse in the sense that I was misdiagnosed and then overmedicated."

Pablo and I discussed several times how this could have happened, but there is no real answer. We have only speculations.

"I've always tried to figure out why, when I ended up in the hospital, why did they misdiagnose me and overmedicate me? Because that'll always remain a mystery. Well, I think I've figured out part of it. I know for one thing, when I arrived there I looked terrible. Just physically looking at me: I hadn't bathed, I had on dirty clothes, I didn't care, disheveled – is that the right word? – and I know, visually, I looked like what you and I think when we see some street people, when we look at them and they're all dirty and all – yeah, I think, 'Looks like someone who's cuckoo.' You know? They're just not in the right world.

"But what went wrong there? Schizophrenia is such a classic catchall. Then I found out something else as to the way the system functions on a legal basis. And here you get into bureaucratic nonsense. If you go in – I don't know how it is today, but – if you go in and are admitted to some psychiatric facility like that, they are by state law bound to make a diagnosis in 78 hours or they have to release you.

"Now that's for the safety of the person. Someone can't just shovel you in. But it leads to a rush in judgment. Because no one – it was *four days* before a professional even talked to me. I was simply put there. Starting to feed you, and here's your room. No one talked to me for four days. By that time they had made their diagnosis on paper, obviously. So, there you have logistical problems with the way the system functions."

Whatever the reason, the result was very close to fatal. Pablo was warehoused in a facility once known as Napa State, completely paralyzed and not expected to recover.

"When I ended up in Napa, they first put me in I-don't-know-how-many different kinds of wards...[The last] was basically a ward where they expected everyone to die... Napa is a great state hospital, but – the overmedication had so severely disrupted the muscular [and] neurological systems that I was catatonic, so that – comatose is a better word – and no muscular ability, I couldn't talk.

"I couldn't do anything for myself. The only muscle that still worked, which was a blessing, was the heart. But nothing else worked. Nothing.

"I could hear, and I could think, but I couldn't speak. So I was on that ward for a good eleven months.

"What happened is much more of an extraordinary type of event than might happen to other people. And medications, I'm all in favor of – when you get them right – medications are very specifically oriented. When you get the wrong medications, are misdiagnosed, it can be devastating. That's the problem there.

"What happened as far as the beginning of recovery is concerned, I remember, they would set me up in a wheelchair all day long, which was very uncomfortable. I couldn't get up on my own. And then at night in one of the blankety-blank hospital beds, which was just ...one night I remember, I couldn't sleep. Talk about patterns of sleep – it was hard to tell the difference between day and night. Because when you're in a hospital room all the time – you're in kind of a twilight zone. You're not [aware] of day or night...When it *was* nighttime, it was very hard to sleep. You're left there just contemplating your own thoughts all the time. And I remember, I was literally by myself – there was no one else there – on this high hospital bed, and there was this *chair*, sitting beside the bed. Just a regular, hospital-type chair. And I remember looking at that chair and I thought, 'You know, I've got nothing else to do, I'd like to get myself into that chair.'

"That was the thought in my mind. And I worked – I had not consciously tried to move. Because for one, it was painful. And I simply couldn't – the brain would say, 'Move your arm,' but the arm wouldn't move. What happened was, it must have been around 10 or 11 – early on – and through the course of the night, I worked all night long, and I got myself into that chair.

"The next morning, when the nurse came to check on her morning duties, she brought my breakfast. She practically dropped the tray and she – I could talk better, then – she said, 'How did you get in the chair?' And I said, 'I did it myself.' She went right out and got the doctor."

Does Pablo hold a grudge? Not particularly. There was a lawsuit, and some money changed hands; but he talks of it in a mild, wondering tone of voice with no real animus. It is just something that happened to him, part of the story of his life. His final comment was, "I must remember, however, that some people end up in institutions and never see the light of day."

Eddie's experience with the system was just as bad in an opposite way. They simply gave up on him, and sent him back out onto the street.

"When I was thrown out of that psychological hospital, they were like, literally, 'We've run out of ideas. And you're screaming and disturbing the other patients.' And then I'm like, 'What if I die out there, because I'm totally hysterical and out of my mind?' And they're like, 'That's an interesting question. We'll have to see.' They just shoved me onto the street with madness just swirling about me. I'm wandering through the streets and everything's two dimensional and coming at me surrealistically, just raging out of my mind and completely out of control, and they say, 'Just fake like it's normal.'

"...I got so *good* at this...So then...then fast-forward because I simply treated myself for 15 years...with various experiments in consciousness. I was so anxious that I was, like, on the verge of going insane when you met me. However, I had learned from Valium how to be that insane, while simultaneously having another part of my brain, which says, 'That's a thing your *body* is doing, because of some other part of your mind. But publicly, you don't have to physically *act like* you're hysterical.' But when you met me, I was completely and utterly hysterical.

"And some people have said, like, they've drove [sic] by, and seen me in a parking lot, and said that spiritual energy...like, they saw me but they weren't hanging out with me but objectively from a distance? They said, 'You just looked like this *soul* in a parking lot, beaming out clouds of energy in every direction.'

"...So what happened is I got gradually healthier."

As you can see, Eddie's viewpoint is pragmatic – but he is not angry, either.

Not all our complaints are against the mental health system. There are plenty of other culprits.

Remember Jessica, the grad student? Who spent ten years getting her Master's? She was deprived of the degree that she had worked for because of her diagnosis:

"The core faculty at my school decided not to put me in Practicum during the time when I could still get three semesters. So I don't get to do my Practicum so I don't get my MFT (Marriage and Family Therapist) degree. And that's a really bad thing that happened because of my disability.

"Which means I could work for a non-profit or maybe even run a non-profit but I can't actually do the individual therapy.

"...they said that – I only had three semesters left at the time, and Practicum is three semesters in a row. And – they didn't approve me for Practicum that semester. Which means I only had two left. Plus there's a financial thing.

"Yeah, that's one of the worst things that happened. After I fucking graduated a Magnum from State...they're not going to approve me."

Shelley told me a long story, which I will reproduce here only in part, of the worst thing that ever happened to her as a result of special chemistry.

"I was raped when I was 19. I was staying in a commune at that time, and I couldn't sleep one night. It was two in the morning, and I couldn't sleep. You know, I can't sleep when people are poking me and pushing me around and there's too many people, so I wanted to get to P---- where there was a house I could sleep in. But it was two a.m. and the only way I had to get there was to hitch.

"So I went out on the highway and put my thumb out, and it was two in the morning and I was *so* Manic. That's why I couldn't sleep, I was Manic. And this guy picked me up; he was a Marine. He was married. And it turned out he was a serial rapist.

"I didn't know this, he drove me, we went to where I needed to go, and I said, 'Hey, that's it, I need to stop here, we're stopping here.' And he said, 'No, you're not.' I heard a click. And all the locks in the car went down.

"I went, *Oh, my god*. He had told me he was this Marine, and he killed a lot of people in Viet Nam, and he had a machete in the back for killing 'gooks,' and I started praying. I started praying, well, Please, don't let me be killed. I was gonna be raped, that was obvious, but please just don't let me be killed …

"He never did any jail time. It was 1971, and they didn't do anything to him. Even though there were five girls including me, right there in a row, that they *knew* about, that he had raped. It was a different time.

"This all happened because I was Manic. When you're manic you have no judgment. That's why I was out on the highway hitching at two a.m. in the morning. I was totally Manic the whole time."

But what's the end of this story? Is she mad? Does she blame him for 'ruining her life'?

She is very happily married to her "third and final husband," as she puts it; they have a spiritual bond that has been going strong for ten years. And when I told her how sad her story made me, she said, "Well, it's a story." And she too advocates forgiveness.

"What does this say?" [she picks up a paper]. "'Dig the dagger out of your heart.' The Dalai Lama said that, and [my husband] wrote that down, 'dig the dagger out of your heart.'"

There are other things to get mad about, of course. There is the way we are seen by society at large. In this matter, we have an extra burden. We are not only disabled, but our disability is invisible. This entails a whole different set of responses. People expect a certain standard of behavior that the invisibly disabled cannot meet. This leads to tensions and misunderstandings.

For instance, I know a psychologist who is legally blind. The difference is not visible – she wears no cane or special glasses. Naturally, she travels by bus, because she can't see well enough to drive. Each time a bus stops in front of her, she has to ask the driver, "Is this the such-and-such bus?" Sometimes they grump at her, "Like it says on the sign, lady. What's wrong with you – you blind or something?" Then she tells them that yes, as a matter of fact, she is legally blind. Now, would they kindly tell her which bus this is? It happens all the time.

Pablo talks about hiding his Obsessive condition in terms of his work, where he would for example often sweep the floor too often or at inappropriate times.

"If you're at work, and your boss sees you doing it and [says], 'What are you doing that for?' they may not know why. But I'm not going to say. Even if you were to turn around and say to someone like that, 'Oh, I'm Obsessive-Compulsive Disorder,' they don't understand."

Short of wearing a sandwich board detailing one's condition, what is one to do? I routinely get stopped at train exits for using my disabled person's card. It is assumed, because I look healthy, that I am a fraud trying to bilk the system. This makes me angry, but my only other choice is to wear the card displayed for everybody to see, and I am vain enough not to want that.

Invisible illnesses cause us to make choices like that. People who don't know better may think you are faking, taking advantage, weak, lazy, demanding, or just plain seeking attention. 'You look OK to me.'

According to *Present Times Journal*, the chronically ill in general are an oppressed population. [2] A long list of stereotypes to which we are subject was generated. Following is a sample.

Sick people are:

-to be pitied
-depressed, hopeless
-not worth anything, aren't productive
-not fully alive
-weak
-contagious (so stay away!)
-fulfilling their bad karma
-a nuisance
-a burden
-unnatural
-ugly…frightening
-unlovable
-babies, dependent

Things we've been told:

-you're not so bad off
-stop complaining
-think of others worse off
-how can you live like that?
-if that happened to me, I'd kill myself
-poor thing
-snap out of it!
-you're just making it worse

---

[2] Reporting on the May 1989 Disability Liberation Workshop.

With this bevy of labels and attitudes to choose from, it is no surprise that the mentally and chronically ill sometimes resent the relatively healthy population around them.

The Worst Things

But the worst things of all are often the things we do to ourselves. Nobody can crush us like we can.

Lisa says:

> "I would have to say that the worst thing that has happened to me is missing so much beauty, so many memories and happy moments because I was trapped inside myself and so miserable there."

Sally squarely blames herself for the stigma she feels.

> "It's made me paranoid. I always think there is something wrong with me with that label. If the breakdowns could be seen as spiritual, without stigma, I'd be happier. But I see I put the stigma on me. No one else does."

Actually Sally's 'worst thing' was inflicted on her by another PASC woman; and it turned into a spiritual opportunity for her.

> "Now that I think of it, the hardest thing that has happened because of all this is I befriended a Bipolar peer who committed suicide. We were friends for four years, became like sisters. She was my poet twin. For a few years after her death I tried to replace her. I can't; the experience has shown me how much of a unique snowflake we all are and each is to be treasured.

"It's been the hardest thing of my life so far. It's also been the fastest transformer of who I am.

"It was so hard at first. But then it got so much – not easier, but more divine. Not that I don't still have insomnia and obsessively think about things at night ever since she left. But everything is more divine, more wonderful, more beautiful. It's sort of a miracle. Because I could have been triggered...gotten really Depressed and done the same thing. But instead it just opened my heart and my soul... It's just been an incredible journey so far.

"...That's probably the biggest miracle of my life, that I got this from her suicide instead of going the other way."

Shanna's 'worst thing' so far (at age 14) might have been her habit of self-mutilation. Yet she did overcome it, and this was partly due to her mother's uncritical acceptance.

"...at the time all that was hidden, that I was all cutting and everything, and Momma didn't know about that yet.

"It was several different reasons. It helped me. I figured...it happened a lot if somebody else hurt me. If somebody else made me angry or something? I figured that was a way to get back at them.

"Until my uncle came. When my uncle came, he found out and told my mom. And my mom was really cool about it. She didn't yell at me or anything. But I was writing at the time, I was writing poetry and stuff, about it, and she

made me read those to her – to get a good idea
[of what I was doing].

"She was really understanding. She
didn't yell at me. She understood, but she did
tell me that I couldn't do it anymore.

"I had impulses to do it, and I wanted to
do it really bad, but I never acted on it, really. I
would think about it, and I would almost do it,
but I never did it really after that. Like I would
still hit stuff after that, but never really full
blown. I never really hurt myself. So, she was
really understanding.

"I haven't done it in I don't know how
long… my mom found out about it and she
helped me out."

She was also helped to stop self-mutilating by
medication, in an indirect way. Early on in her treatment, she
was put briefly on Haldol.

"Everybody I've talked to about that
says Haldol is the worst to put a kid on.
Momma says it's a sedatement [sic], it sedates
you. I was out of it for a long time. I didn't
think about cutting for a long time because I
was so out of it."

Ultimately, Shanna feels she has benefited from going
through these experiences.

"Me and Momma were talking one day,
and she said, 'Gee. If I could, I would take it for
you,' take my stress and stuff. I told her, 'I'd
rather you not,' pretty much, because it made
me more understanding. I tell myself, if I had
not had Bipolar Disorder, I wouldn't

understand people having suicidal thoughts, or having certain things wrong with them. I would have just said, 'Oh, you're nuts. Get away from me.' But now that I've been through it, pretty much, I'm like, 'I've been through it, talk to me.'"

How to Forgive

How do we get around the hostility caused by very real grievances? How do we make our way to the humility and forgiveness required by the Eighth Step?

For me, it helps enormously to remember how ignorant 'standard chemistry' people are. This is just a fact, and not always their fault. With the best vocabulary in the world, one still cannot describe what it is actually like to have, say, a psychotic break. Even the most creative and imaginative friends will not understand, though they may *think* they do. To have your mind malfunction is an experience like no other. It cannot be had second hand.

I once had a brother who died of AIDS. One of the things he went through towards the end was an episode of delirium.

We had discussed my special chemistry before. I had done my best to share the experience; and as a wordsmith, I think I did a pretty fair job. But after his delirium, Mark told me, "I thought I understood what you meant. But I didn't. I didn't get it at all."

It really is not possible to make someone see inside your head. People have been trying from the beginning of time, and all we have come up with are hundreds and thousands of philosophies and religions, many of which won't even acknowledge each other. Police can tell you, too, that even eyewitness accounts are never exactly the same.

Here's the problem: every human being has his or her own reality. There are as many realities as there are people in the world.

Some of us share a lot of basic material, but no two minds are identical. And if something is not in your reality, you *cannot* react to it appropriately. It's not that you don't want to, you *can't*. You just don't know what you don't know.

And that's the crux of the matter. These folks wouldn't be so cruelly stupid if they had ever been in our shoes. But they haven't. It is for us to make allowances for them. Even the courts recognize the difference between 'murder' and 'manslaughter.' The difference is *intent*. If people *do not know* what they are doing, we can't blame them in the same way.

Also, there is the matter of practicality. If you wish to join the fight to change stigma, more power to you. But in the meanwhile, this is the way the world is. There may be millions of us, but we are still a minority. It is much better to cultivate a water-off-the-back philosophy than to walk around in a red haze of rage. A self-comforting, cushioning attitude will go a long way toward preserving your nerves.

As they once said on Saturday Night Live, "It is easier to wear slippers than to carpet the whole world."

Forgiveness is a strange beast. Some folks seem born to dispense it as easily as rain. Others hold smoldering grudges for decades, and this seems to be part of their temperamental makeup.

To them I say: think what you are doing to your body. Think what you are doing to what's left of your nervous system. If you are holding onto anger and pain, keeping them alive, blowing on the embers lovingly in hopes of someday getting adequate revenge, getting 'justice' – forget it. In the short term of one lifetime, often there is no justice. Whether there is a greater justice in some longer-term sense is a matter for religions to wrangle over.

Besides, is it really justice that we want? Or are we waiting for yesterday to change? Are we waiting for the world somehow to turn back around as if 'it' had never happened? And when do we wise up?

What we are for sure doing is producing burning, chronic stress in ourselves. As Lily Tomlin once put it, "Lady, you are making bad weather inside your body." And it is entirely pointless. We are never going to be able to hurt those people in the same way, to the exact same degree, as they hurt us. What we are doing is comparable to locking ourselves up in an Iron Maiden, yelling as the nails sink into us, "This will show them!"

It won't. Sorry.

Forgiveness consists, as far as I can determine, of perspective. Emotional distance, regardless of distance in time or space, is the key. As long as the unfair action is still giving us pain, we cannot let it go. As long as we see what happened as personal and deliberate, we will continue to feel that pain. As long as we reject who we are now, instead of incorporating what happened into our personality and moving on, just so long are we stuck on the point of impact. As far as our heart is concerned, it happened yesterday. As long as we consider our lives ruined, they are.

Therapy was designed to take the ache out of this. Living the event over in a diary or with a friend or counselor can eventually help us separate from what happened. We can start to see the perpetrators as flawed or sick or stupid, not personifications of evil. In time, we can come to see whatever hurt us as something finished, done with, no longer part of our daily lives. Even if we are still dealing with the consequences, we can approach it rationally (How do I work this?) rather than passionately (She ruined my life!), and get much better results.

The key is to let go of the point of impact and focus on getting results. *Your life matters. What you do with it matters. How you got here does not.*

Short of natural disaster, most of our hurts are caused simply by the same old weak, silly, narrow-minded people we all are sometimes. Just people. Even the biggest 'system' is made up merely of human beings. And for human beings, who are so complex and fragile, we have to make allowances.

If you really can't forgive – and who knows, maybe some things shouldn't be forgiven – then I would advise you to put it aside for the purposes of this Step. What hurt you is important, but you can't let it keep you sick. Imagine putting all your resentments into a fortified trunk from which even radiation can never leak, and throw it somewhere hard to get to – the bottom of the Mariana Trench, say. Get it temporarily out of the way. It can only keep you from doing your job.

I don't mean any of us should turn into doormats. I don't mean we should let the same folks hurt us again and again. Injustice and unfairness must certainly be opposed. But not right this minute. Put it all aside. Breathe deeply.

Then go to work.

What We Did To Them

Let's not forget the things we've done that have hurt other people. Yes, you were the one most hurt. But if your house burned to the ground, and also destroyed the top story of your neighbors' house, wouldn't you show a little sympathy – if only out of courtesy? After all, it was YOUR fire. It's true we couldn't control our actions. That's why we forgive ourselves. But other people still have to live with the consequences of our actions, whether we meant to do it or not.

Some of us have racked up some terrific debt, quite literally. During Manic sprees, Bipolar PASCs can rack up tremendous debt well beyond their ability to pay – ever. Here is Shelley's story:

> "I've done bankruptcy. I've lost $62,500 down the toilet. What was it, 11 years ago?... Lost. $62,500 worth of credit card debt. For $700 I paid the guy – you know, here you go, $700 – He's one of the last Commies. 'This is an act of revolution, you know!'...

> "You could do that for $700 back then. ...I can't remember, some Jewish guy, really radical with long hair and a beard, down on Montgomery Street. And I remember he only wanted $700, so I paid cash, seven one-hundred-dollar bills...He said, 'Well, sign a few things, what do you have?' Nothing. 'Oh, you're on SSI? Great, great. Great, great, great, you have nothing.' Badadadadada. 'Here, sign on the dotted line,' 17,000 places. So I signed.

And six, eight months later, 'show up at this court.' And da-DUH! There was like a whole bunch of people there, it was like this big mass wedding! Yeah, it was jolly, it was fun. And I was down [whispering] sixty-two-five. That's quite a sum. And Ka-CHING! DOWN THE TOILET!"

She has also done a lot of damage over the years to her home and possessions:

> "See, the reason I haven't been in mental institutions is because I've always had a man around me to just, like, do this to me [she demonstrates by putting her arms around herself] hold me in a straitjacket so I'm wiggling, I'm wiggling, I'm, like, wriggling – I want to – AGH! I want to take everything, I want to just take everything and [she mimes throwing] – my Macintosh, I won't do that to that, because I know I won't be able to put that back together. But otherwise I'll just wreck the place. You know, like, if I get crazy. Then I have to spend the whole day, like, putting it together – I hate that.

> "Look what I've done! Dammit!"

That's a lot of amends to make.

Or there is the damage done by the things we say during episodes of sickness. Shelley describes it graphically:

> "I was...to the point of 'I'm gonna kill you!' You know, I've said that to people that I love! 'I'm gonna claw your eyes out! I'm gonna kill you! I need to rip all your furniture apart.' I mean, I've done really wild things."

Not to mention how much we asked of our partners; how much they paid for our special requirements. Eddie Smith's needs were rather unique:

> "By the time I met Annie...I said, 'Here's the deal. You can't date me the way a normal person does. I have to have a separate bed. Plus, me driving you crazy, plus me seeing that I'm driving you crazy, 'cause I'm up all night, will drive *me* crazy. So you have to sleep in a separate bed.

> "'When we're on dates together, if I tell you the date has to end because I'm becoming so claustrophobic that I'm going to go insane, then we have to end our date.

> "'Um, I'm incapable of bonding close enough to feel faithful. You have to let me, like, make out with other chicks. Or I'll go insane. If I'm trapped. You can't *live* near me. You have to live 10 blocks over at least.'

> "And there was just this list of mad shit. And for whatever the fuck reason, which now to me makes no sense, she just signed on to the whole deal."

After a while, the question is not, "What have we done to them?" It's, "Why do we still have anyone at all?"

The Twelve-Step system requires that we not let these things just sit there and stink. We must go to the person we hurt and admit that we were wrong, and do something that *they* will consider an adequate repayment for their pain.

So after we've identified the harmful things we did in regards to special chemistry (the Eighth Step), we have to go on to the Ninth: making amends.

Making Amends

The process doesn't have to be terribly complicated. Sometimes we just ask what they want in amends and they'll tell us.

We tell the person what diagnosis we have, and explain that we had no control over what we did. We make it clear that we are sorry they were hurt. If there are losses such as money or property involved, we replace it or pay for it if we can. Then we let the matter go – even if they don't get it or don't forgive us.

Unfortunately we cannot promise never to do it again. We are still not in control of our unusual chemistry. But we can outline the drugs/therapies we are using. We can promise to stay with our therapy. We can promise to try.

The important thing about amends is that we must think of the other person's needs, not ours. The point is to try to give them back what we took: their pride, if we embarrassed them; their self-respect, if we humiliated them; and so forth. Some people may need to know that we still love them. Different people have different needs.

For instance, my first husband was a very proud Middle Eastern man. His concern, often stated, was that he couldn't control my behavior. He felt he ought to be able to. Husbands control their wives in his culture. His relatives accused him, too. Why couldn't he make me behave in a stable manner? Why couldn't he stop my impulsive, unwise actions? He was my husband, wasn't he? That was his job, wasn't it? As he saw it, he had somehow failed as a man. He was humiliated.

So in my letter to him (it would have been dangerous at that time to confront him in person), I explained simply that it turned out I had been ill, mentally ill, and nobody knew it, not even me. There was nothing that could change that, it was permanent, *and there was nothing he could have done to fix it*. This let him off the hook in his area of deepest concern. It was not necessary to explain about pills, genetics, or therapy. It was not necessary to mention the many valid issues that had torn us apart. It was not my business, in that letter, to apportion blame or to explain everything away or even to be right. It was not my job to tell him what he did wrong. There was a time and place for that, but not now. It was my job to relieve him where he hurt most.

The next time I saw him, he invited me into a coffee shop and bought a cookie for me and my mother. Only four years prior, he had been stalking me!

Relieve their hurt. This is the goal.

Sometimes this may take money, if that was how we hurt them.

It will be important when we make amends to know about our own chemistry. We need to be able to explain in a simple, straightforward way what was going on. People have a right to know that. People need to know that we didn't treat them badly because we hated or disrespected them, or because we didn't care. It was because we were sick. This is part of the healing we offer – letting them know our actions were not personal.

We ought to know about our own condition in any case. If we haven't before, we might want to bone up now. We don't have to be rocket scientists. We don't have to study the exchange of neurotransmitters in the brain, or the reproductive odds of genes. There are plenty of simple, free brochures from the National Institute of Mental Health, or articles from popular magazines. Just go see your librarian. Or google it.

These can give us an overall idea of how our particular illness works. So we will be able to say, "Remember when I did so-and-so? Here's why that happened."

What Happens Next

Ultimately, what happens next is none of our business. Once we have done our best to make up for our blunders, we are through.

It helps, though, to be prepared: we may get a negative response. They may think we are talking a lot of hogwash. Or they may not *care* what our reasons were. They may prefer to continue being hurt or angry, or not want to see us. That is their privilege. Try not to be too upset by this. When damage has been done, sometimes it can't be fixed. When people see us behaving badly, they believe we chose that behavior. They may not be able to comprehend that we honestly couldn't help it.

And even if they do understand, they still may choose not to stick around for part two. That is a judgment call our friends have to make on their own, and they have the right to make it.

Here again is where forgiveness and letting go is needed. Despite our best efforts, they may never get it. They may never buy the disease theory at all, or understand it, or care. If they blame us, however, we must decline to blame ourselves.

Give yourself credit for trying, and go on. Not everything that breaks can be repaired.

But you have flexed some crucial spiritual muscles in making the attempt.

And you'll be amazed at what expansive relief you will feel. Relief from guilt (and possibly mended relationships) are healthy things for people with our built-in emotional burdens. We feel saner: we can face the world with our shoulders a lot straighter.

That, of course, is the ultimate point.

Outer Tips for Inner Peace

Strategy 8: Coupling Up

One of the things you may be thinking is that you'll never have a good relationship again.

Bunk. Humans are extremely complex. There are people out there who need exactly what you have to offer, no matter how strange the package deal. Trust me on this.

If you're already in a relationship when you get your diagnosis, you may be afraid to lose it.

Well, yeah, that might happen. I won't lie.

It all depends on the terms of the relationship. Every couple has a set of *agreements*, whether stated or not. Some agree that they will stick together no matter what. Some agree that they will part in the morning. Some partners have the agreement that one (or both) will have sex with other partners. Some even agree that one will beat up the other. Like I said, there are all kinds out there. We have no idea why they need some of the things they do – and it's not our business. It's a matter of free choice.

Here's the thing about agreements: If one of you *changes the terms* mid-stream, sometimes the partnership doesn't last.

But if you go into the relationship with the understanding that one of you already has a heart problem, or epilepsy, or a PASC condition, or is in a wheelchair, the other partner *knows* that special care will be needed and accepts that ahead of time.

It is entirely possible to find such partners. I have, many times. You will find that you have better luck with compassionate people, men and women who already know that PASC is a health condition, not a character defect. You may, as I have, find better luck among creative types. People who relish differences instead of fearing them are a good bet.

Strategy 9: Rules of PASC Relationships

1) <u>Tell your partner before substantial commitment is made</u>, but not so early that they don't even know you yet! This is not first-date material.

2) <u>Be the best partner you can be</u>. This is a lifelong endeavor. Even if we are married, we must try to improve what kind of partners we are. Strive to be a better communicator, a better friend, a pleasant companion, a fun bed partner. If most of the time we are terrific to be with, our lovers can put up with a few hardships.

I can't tell you in this small section how to be a better person – but I think you know, anyway. All of us know areas where we could improve.

3) <u>Always work on your sanity</u>. People will put up a lot more cheerfully with someone who is *trying* to be sane than someone who doesn't care. If we are working on our treatment, going to therapy, improving our personal and spiritual lives, they will be more inclined to stay. That goes for friends and employers, too.

4) <u>Try not to take your symptoms out on your partner</u>. Sad to say, sometimes we are going to have to fake. Yes, I mean 'acting normal' when we don't feel it. I don't mean fool a doctor or get away with something bad. I mean when we are starting to get a little off, but there is no way to escape our company or our job or our partner for awhile yet, we need to do our best to act normal and polite, even as we are trying to get away to somewhere safe. If this means admitting we're in poor shape and asking to be excused, we do this. But we do it politely.

I found the hardest thing to 'fake' was tone of voice. I could manage the polite words, but the rage (or whatever) would slip through and spoil the whole show. I remember once loudly shouting, "NO!" to a co-worker when she asked if I wanted some help. Then I saw the hurt on her face. It wasn't her fault I was full of irrational rage. She was just in the wrong place at the wrong time. I made some excuse about having a really bad headache, but she never trusted me after that, and I never felt good around her. That's when I understood that using neutral *words*, all by itself, was just not enough.

Until then I had believed that just picking acceptable words – things that would have sounded fine on paper, with no inflection – ought to be good enough for people. It was hard just to do that! My mind was running away, my emotions were exploding. The world was barely there for me. If I just went through the proper motions, they should be satisfied. I couldn't pretend to a happy attitude. Jesus, I was in hell! What did they want, blood? They were asking too much.

Now I understand how deeply people count on tone of voice, facial expression, body language. It conveys at least half of the message, if not more. You can start a fight or ruin a relationship, by the wrong intonation at a critical time.

If you can't fake it, you must get out of there. Say something, anything, "I'm not well, I need to go lie down." Whatever. But if you're going to hang in till the end of the conversation, the workday, the evening out, you need to learn to act a little. For their sakes.

Not everybody will appreciate this. Not everybody will buy it. Someone I know was once unkind enough to tell me he'd overheard a table of acquaintances discussing me. They complained I was not 'genuine,' my smile was not 'real.' I wasn't sincere, they said.

Yeah, sometimes. It was true, and it hurt me to hear it.

But I reminded myself that I was still doing the best thing for everybody. Those women at that table would be the first to complain if I screamed out what I really felt! So I have to disregard that input. You can't please everyone. Period. Part of the art of manners is that people should not *know* it is an effort.

I know this does not sound appealing. But think about it: do you really want to scare or embarrass your friends and drive them away? Do you really want to make scenes in coffee houses? How do you wish to be viewed?

You can be the crazy, scary lady down the street if you want to. That's the other option. But there's a price for that, too.

5) <u>Remember you are valuable</u>. Do NOT fall for thinking you are 'damaged' and can only be around 'damaged' people. This will only net you someone who can't come through when the chips are down. You will eventually find people – normal people – who enjoy your quirky turn of mind, or who like nurturing the sensitive and moody. Or they simply find you worthwhile! Can you deal with that?

But be reasonable. If we are in the early days of our treatment, we may be best alone. If our pills don't work yet, if our lives are in chaos, if we go psychotic three times a week, we do not yet have much to offer to a partner.

The key word is 'yet.' Work on yourself. The rest will come.

Step Ten

Take Stock Regularly

"Continued to take personal inventory,
and when we were wrong, promptly admitted it."

- adapted from the Twelve Steps of AA

"The wise have always known that no one can make much of his life until self-searching becomes a regular habit..."

-*Twelve Steps and Twelve Traditions*

Step Ten

There are basically three types of inventory that should become a regular part of our lives as Twelve-Step workers. One is the exhaustive, once-a-year process we have gone over in Step Four (some do this more than once a year, whenever they feel they need it). Then there is the spot-check inventory to take at moments of turmoil, when we question our anger, for instance, and try to show some self-restraint before flailing out in all directions. These should become routine parts of the way we operate.

Thirdly, we are recommended to take an inventory each evening, to give ourselves a fair picture of how we have done that day. It's a chance to see what we might like to change tomorrow.

Amends become easier the faster we catch them. It's a lot easier to apologize for last week than for something from 10 years ago (especially if you haven't spoken since then!).

How all this relates to being PASC is very simple. I suggest that before going to sleep we add one question: *How sane was I today?*

This is not a golden chance to criticize ourselves. It is to help us get a picture of how we are handling life's problems. Did we deal with them rationally? Did something push us over the edge today? What was it? Maybe amends will be due for something said in a PASC-related rage. Maybe we were burdened with Paranoia and accused a friend of something. Maybe we were so Depressed we stood somebody up rather than leave the bed.

It is like taking our mental temperature. And if we are very, very lucky and careful, we may find clues to prevent some problems in the first place.

Some we can't. I'm not turning about-face and suggesting we can 'control' our disease. I am suggesting that there are a few methods of prevention. Sometimes there are warning signs that can give us time to get out of range of trouble. I am suggesting that we *might* learn to identify our triggers and avoid them.

This may not be the case with you. Some mental symptoms simply happen with no warning. But if you think that from time to time there are clues that happen first, it may be worth examining. Ask yourself, what happened just before the episode? Were there any hints? Are there physical sensations, or emotional feelings, that are typical when I am about to go off-base? *Can I learn to see this coming?*

And if I can, what should I do about it? Call my doctor? Take a pill? Go away from public places until it passes?

Pay attention as often as you can. Keep trying to trace it back. What happened just before I became out of control? What were the circumstances, the place? Who was there? Do they always have that effect on you? Was it crowded and noisy and distracting? Was it too, too silent and depressing? Was I hungry and tired? What was the weather like?

Um, the weather? Well, yes. For myself, I eventually found that bright direct sunlight or excessive heat were a direct cause of my worst states of mind. Certain states of mind led to rage, psychosis, and The Voice (supposedly) of God in my head. (I know it's not really God because of the STUPID things it says.)

Now, I wear sunhats, always walk on the shady side of the street, and keep my sunglasses on. If I have been out too long and feel that grim, tight feeling in the head coming on, I get to a cool, private place as soon as humanly possible. It's saved me a lot of painful scenes. I haven't heard the Voice in…what? A decade? Almost never are strangers subjected to my irrational rage. Even my intimates hardly ever get anything but the earliest stages (hostility and irritation). I have learned to head it off at the pass. I just don't go there any more.

It's possible that you can do this, too. Try to recognize the early states of mind, the feelings before it all goes tilted. Not just emotions, but physical feelings, too. Our bodies can often be the first to know. Are there certain phrases or tones of voice you tend to use? Certain clothes that you wear on Depressed days? How does your stomach feel, and your neck? Maybe there are certain people that you only want to be around when you are not quite yourself. I notice that when things are getting bad for me, I want to smoke, though I quit years ago. Does it happen under certain kinds of stress, such as hurry or too much noise or in large pushy crowds? Perhaps you can limit your exposure to these things.

Or, as I once suggested, use other humans as our bellwether. When it seems everybody starts objecting to everything we say or do, or actively trying to stop us, we may have slipped over the line. If a whole roomful of people seems embarrassed or shocked, if strangers are staring at us one after another, we may have tipped too far. This is not the time to be stubborn. This is the time to pause and question ourselves. It is very mentally healthy, and one of the program's axioms, to ask whether the one who's out of line is us.

If we can't stop this time, that's OK. We can take note for next time. Where, exactly, did we lose control? What happened between the last time we felt OK and the time we knew we'd lost it? Are there any clues there? Any patterns? Definitely look for patterns. Things that happen over and over are things to steer clear of.

Please note that none of this 'avoidance' advice is aimed at people whose problem is Anxiety or Agoraphobia. If a fear-based reaction is your problem, then the more often you can confront the scary situation and walk through it, the better off you are. You need to experience, over and over, that if you do the feared thing, feel the feared feelings, NOTHING BAD HAPPENS. Fear is crippling. Give in to it, and pretty soon you won't have a life. In cases of irrational Anxiety, head into it rather than away from it. This is a different kind of problem with a different treatment.

After we have practiced careful monitoring of triggers for a long time, we may more and more often be able to say, at the end of the day, "Yes, I was sane. No, I hurt no one. Yes, I had a bad moment: and here is what I did about it."

Give yourself huge credit for that. In this business, trying counts for a whole lot. We may not be able to 'stop' the insanity – but maybe, just maybe, we can catch it at baby size. Maybe, just maybe, we can keep it private. Maybe, over time, there will be fewer and fewer amends to make.

And it can be a lifesaver.

Learning your Limits

Learning your limits may be the most important thing you do to live a relatively 'normal' life. Like a person with any serious condition, such as a heart problem, there are going to be things you can no longer do.

Obviously, being PASC will change your life in many ways. One of the ways, I suggest, is that you must *slow down*. Haste and pressure and deadlines cause stress, and one of our new limits is that we cannot take a great deal of stress without coming apart. Of course there are stressors in every life. But we can cut them down right away by cutting down the pace.

It is just not smart to schedule one appointment after another (and then 10 chores plus quality family time) on any given day. We will get overwhelmed and sick, and we will act out. At least, I have found it so. There is a certain craziness that comes with too much stimulation (this is one reason, perhaps, why many PASC patients prefer to live alone). There is a certain craziness endemic to never sitting back to relax, to enjoy our time for what it is – a very precious commodity.

Build your schedule around your greatest weakness, so that things can still run reasonably well if you become incapacitated. Arrange someone in advance whom you can count on to take care of the pets, or the cooking. Make sure your appointments are somewhat flexible, so that people know it depends upon your health (this does not apply to appointments with, say, Medicare or SSDI; they are notoriously rigid). This way your friends will know, if you have to cancel, that they are not being stood up. I am not saying 'be a flake'. I am saying that you need to allow some room in your life for the unexpected.

I suggest you be careful about commitments and promises. It may be a while before you are reliable again, even to yourself. Tell your friends, "I'd like to come, but it depends on my health." Or, "I'll be there if I can," or, "Thanks for telling me; I'll have to see." You may not know what state you are in until an hour before the appointment. If you swore up and down you'd come – and bring all the beer besides – and then just don't show up, you are going to get unpopular. People will stop inviting you anywhere. You don't have to be a flake just because you are PASC. If they know you're doing your best – hey, they don't have to know what the problem is! – you will still be getting invitations when the day comes that your condition becomes more predictable.

Schedule around your weaknesses. For instance, I have enough Depression that I am almost incapable of getting up in the morning. So I schedule all appointments for afternoon. If I have an important meeting I leave a chunk of free time afterward, to regroup my energies and get centered again. I never schedule more than two (or *maybe* three) events in one day – in fact, I often can't make a third one. If I need to put something off, I do so, unless the deadline is truly inflexible (i.e. term paper due dates or court dates). My to-do list tends to be short, and if I get to anything past the third item, it's gravy. Most things can wait, if they have to, because *nothing is more important than my mental health.* And I do mean *nothing*.

Let people think I'm lazy if they want to. What counts is that I am not in a straitjacket.

Depending on the type of symptoms you have, build your own time patterns. But don't try to be a superhero. Nothing will happen if the grass doesn't get mowed today. This is a particularly important thing for the Anxiety-prone to remember.

Another practice that helps is doing *only one thing at a time*. As special chemistry people, our brains have got way too much to handle. It only snarls things up to be multi-tasking. Whatever you are doing, I recommend doing *just that*. Some people would call this Zen, I suppose. It is an extension of the

'One Day at a Time' principle that recovering alcoholics use. Don't be thinking about all the other things you have to do, or trying to do several at once. That will make for a mess.

Or a car wreck. Driving a car is one of the most heavy multi-tasking activities we do, which is why I tell people NOT to drive if they are feeling at all disturbed. Even in a short distance you could lose your right front fender or your life, not to mention the wear and tear you are putting on other people's nerves and property.

Here is another Anxiety-relieving trick I use. A little thing you might try is keeping an endless to-do list of *everything* that comes to your mind to be done. It doesn't matter if this list is miles long and contains really low priority projects you won't get to for months. The idea is to get it *off your mind*. You don't have to worry that you'll forget it. You wrote it down. You can look it up any time. This is not so much about organization as about keeping your mind clear. Relaxing.

The other advantage of a list like this is for days when you feel blah, bad, or just not very functional. It's not too much fun to just stare at the wall and smoke. And as years pass, when you look back on your life, you won't want to be treated to an endless vista of pain and boredom and brooding. On days like this, you can take out your endless list, and find one of those low-priority mindless tasks that is just enough to keep you busy, but doesn't require much thinking. You will feel better about yourself that way. You are going to lose too many days in your life to mental illness as it is.

Of course, if it's just a day when you truly *cannot* function, then you don't have to do anything. That's what TV is for.

To summarize: know the onset of your symptoms, if you can. When you sense you're in the danger zone, stop. Take an antipsychotic, or whatever is appropriate. Then go home and rest if possible, till the danger has passed. Keep your life simple, and keep it slow.

At work, this can be a problem. I restrain myself to 19 hours a week maximum, and never put myself in a critical or leadership position. Intrigue and pressure and politics are not good for me. I make sure somebody above me knows my condition, so there is someone to give me permission to break for a while and go lie down in the employee lounge if I get unstable. Some people may talk about me, but those in the know are impressed that they never have to see me blow up or 'act crazy'. And if you have to go home – well, you do. Be their best employee except for the glitches in your attendance, and they probably will keep you anyway. I worked this way in libraries for 12 years.

Handling Psychosis

I don't like scare tactics, but I need to warn you. Becoming psychotic in public is not just embarrassing and messy – it can be dangerous.

We need to understand this: *out of control people are scary. When people are scared, they do extreme things.*

When we are psychotic, people don't know what we're thinking, they can't figure out what we'll do. If they call the police, we may be in deep trouble. The police might not talk to us gently and ask who our doctor is. They might just wonder if we are dangerous and get out their guns. We could end up in jail, or shot, or dead, *even if we are harmless.*

It happens. Somebody imprisoned in their own private hell waves a pocket knife, or even a butter knife. Maybe in his reality, someone is coming to kill him. Or maybe he never even hears them telling him to put up his hands and lie down slowly. Maybe he reaches for a piece of paper in his pocket, and they think it's a weapon. People get shot for things like that. I'm sorry, but it's true.

It is a really, really bad idea to stick around in public if we have reason to believe we are leaving the common reality.

Be sure anyone you live with knows what to do. You can tell them you have Post Traumatic Stress Disorder if you don't want to cop to mental illness. Just make sure they know to call your doctor, or your therapist, or the hospital, or your best friend, but *not the police.* Post the numbers somewhere handy. Psychotic breaks are going to happen, but *you cannot afford to have them in public!* I'm telling you – go somewhere safe. SAFE means someplace where you won't bother anyone, and they won't bother you. Don't come unglued in front of strangers if you can help it.

If you feel yourself losing it, reach for your anti-psychotics (you have them on you, right?). The next thing, if you can't get home fast, is to get to a hospital or at least somewhere you can be left alone for awhile.

What do you do after that? NOTHING.

I am quite serious.

No matter what you feel, hear, or see, don't do *anything* and don't say *anything*. You can't hurt anybody by being silent. You might offend someone, I suppose, or get sent to a hospital, but you won't be seen as a threat. They can't punish you for being kind of comatose.

This may sound like odd advice, but it comes from decades of experience. If we start acting on anything at all when we are psychotic, there is no telling where it will lead. We are not in control. The only safe thing to do is nothing. Train yourself to be still and quiet like a small animal hiding in the weeds while a predator passes by.

It works. Forget about danger, for a minute…let's just talk about human relations. We can't say the one unforgivable thing if we don't talk. We can't alienate every friend we ever had by just sitting still. We can't throw our fists through the wall if we're not moving. We just take our pill, and then wait for it to kick in.

Do nothing. If you wait, it will pass. These attacks do not last forever. *Nothing* lasts forever. And we can't be jailed or divorced or prosecuted or embarrassed by something we didn't do. (I suppose we could get jailed for not answering the police, if it comes to that – but what does it matter whether we sit silently in an alley or in a jail cell?)

I had a vivid experience of how this works just a few nights ago. Never mind how it happened – I allowed myself to get pushed too hard, and I snapped.

But just before I snapped, I told my husband, "I am **this close** to losing it completely!!!" And I took my maximum dose of anti-psychotics and lay down.

It is hard for me to describe what happened next. A wave of fury and hatred swept over me such as I have never known. It was so huge, so compelling, all I could do was lie there and feel it. It took everything I had just to BE STILL. The hatred broke over me like a monstrous tidal wave, and I just let it break.

I did think a few coherent things. I thought, "This is how Hitler felt." I thought, "This is how murderers feel." I thought, "This is how fathers feel when they beat their children." I also thought of things to say. I wanted to spit the poison out in the worst way. But I remembered the one thing I knew absolutely: *This will pass. If you don't do anything, you won't be sorry.*

And it did pass. It had broken over me like a huge wave and swallowed me alive. But then, like a wave, it drained away and left me behind, a little rock on the sand. I was rational again, I was 'me' again, and all I could think was, "Thank God I didn't do anything. Thank God I didn't say anything."

After that my husband (whom I do *not* hate, though I had only seconds ago) waited quietly until I spoke, and we talked softly of what had happened and what I might do to work on this in the future.

If you are overwhelmed by feelings, or voices, or anything wild, be still. Be quiet. It will pass.

If it doesn't, sooner or later you will have to go to the hospital.

Which is OK. It's safe there. That's the whole point.

Mood Disorders 101

Your emotions can also be symptoms, which makes it tricky.

I would say that any time a feeling comes up that seems huge and overwhelming and it sweeps you away and you *must* act---BE SUSPICIOUS!!! If it feels THAT big it is probably a chemical surge and you should ride it out as quietly as humanly possible. Don't speak yet. Incredible harm can be done in only a few minutes if you give in to this stuff.

The trick is to find some safe way to release the excess emotional energy. This is a very important thing to learn!

Emotion is a tangible form of energy that *must be used in some way before it will disperse.* This is what therapists are trying to say when they advise you not to stuff away your feelings. There may or may not be some real issue or cause buried in your emotion. But you won't know until you have siphoned the excess energy off! Run for blocks, or scream into a pillow, or in the locked cab of your car, or somewhere the neighbors won't hear you. Take a shovel and attack the most stubborn weeds on the block. Anything that will *physically* dispel the energy without harming live people is valid.

Talking or writing about it may not be enough. One thing I have found I can be sure of when it comes to emotion is that I will always have too much of it, not too little. Don't count to ten – count to 300, while digging through a rock wall with your bare hands!

Afterwards, when you are human and rational again, you might find you still have a real beef with someone. Then you can discuss it.

Other Tips

To avoid over-stress, we may have to avoid fights and raised voices. They can escalate into horrendous scenes. Practice saying, "We'll talk about this later; right now I'm too upset." Use that line as often as you have to. *Walk away from the drama.* Then go take a long walk, or do whatever centers you and gives you perspective. When I have failed to do this, I have made The Scene From Hell. It solved nothing. It's not worth it. And as I said, it's dangerous.

The other thing you will have to do – and it's hard – is learn your economic limits. You cannot afford to be in heavy debt. Don't use your credit card except for emergencies. You don't need to be paying Master Charge $300 a month when your monthly income is $600.

It's hard to live within such small limits. I didn't do it right myself. Oh, I paid all my bills and never went to the movies. My entertainment was library books and old vinyl records and friends on the telephone. But I was addicted to fashionable clothes, and had a reputation for giving terrific gifts. So when my husband married me, he was suddenly saddled with $17,000 in debt.

Isn't that a pretty wedding present?

He paid it off, like the prince he is – a gift which I did not ask for. But I will be paying it back to him for – who knows, decades? I don't have to, he said it was a gift, but I'm going to, because otherwise I just can't live with myself. And I am the lucky one-in-a-million who found a White Knight. What are your chances? Really?

If this money trouble sounds like you – or if you had debt before all this happened – you can attend the free meetings of Debtors Anonymous. They have a great program and offer a lot of help.

A few final hints: As I've said, mental illness can cause a lot of chaos in your life. You should at least make sure that you have a few basic things at *all* times: your keys, your wallet, the name and number of your doctor, *and your medications*.

Here's the drill: Write on a card or a slip of paper the name of every medication you take, what dose, and how often. Like this:

XYZ Pill: 4 mg. Twice daily.
ABC Pill: 1 mg. At bedtime.

Be sure you list them all. On the bottom or on the top, write the name of your doctor and his/her phone number. Put that in your wallet. Leave it in there all the time.

Now: decide where you are going to keep your wallet and keys forever from now on. I know that may sound silly. But if you are sliding in and out of reality, you need to have **habits that your body does automatically**. *Always* put your wallet in the same pocket or compartment of your purse. *Always* put it on the same space on the table when you are home. Do the same with your keys. Once your body gets used to putting it there automatically, you will *always* be able to find your wallet and keys, no matter what state your mind is in. And if there is an emergency and you are found unconscious, the police will *always* know whom to call, and the doctors will *always* know what to give you. Even if you can't tell them. (And you will never again have to roam around the house saying, "Where the hell did I put my keys?" while your wife laughs.)

I want to pass on one more thing to you. When I was in Alcoholics Anonymous, somebody very wisely told me: "It doesn't matter if you have to act like a jerk, just stay sober!" That saved me, lots of times. So I want to adapt that for you: Act like a jerk if that's what it takes, but stay sane! Like, let's say you promised to bring all the beer for that fictional party I mentioned. But at the last minute you realize that you are totally on the verge of psychosis and need to stay in the house. SO STAY IN THE HOUSE. Yeah, maybe your friends will think you are an utter creep for not showing up with the beer. SO WHAT? Be an utter creep, but don't show up and throw a scene that will ruin the party for everyone and end with you in a squad car. They can live without you for one evening, and there will be other parties.

Sanity *first*. That's the single best piece of advice I know.

So there you are. Learn your limits. Stick to them.

Then more and more often, at the end of the day when you ask yourself, "Was I sane today?" the answer will be "Yes."

Outer Tips to Inner Peace

Strategy 10: Don't Drive Disturbed

Do I need to tell you that it's not a good idea to drive psychotic? Or even just kind of on the edge?

I've done it. I don't recommend it. Once, I got pulled over and sent to a hospital: police cars, ambulance and all. Another time, too fragile to handle the pressures of rush hour, I beat my head on the steering wheel and screamed. I wouldn't give the wheel to any of my passengers. They were not happy.

Not an ideal situation.

Another time, I did something weird or rude at a gas pump – I honestly don't remember what – and the people in the opposite car started hassling me. I felt hostile, so I pulled out my big conversation stopper. "I'm mentally ill!" I barked. "Don't mess with me!"

One of them hollered incredulously, "If you're crazy, man, what are you doing on the road?"

I scowled and burned rubber out of the station. *'Oh, that would be just great!'* I told myself. *'Imagine if they took away the driving privileges of everyone with a diagnosis!"*

But a few miles later a little clarity clicked on in my head. *"They're right. I'm a mess. What AM I doing on the road?"*

It's dangerous to everyone when we get behind the wheel less than sane. For one thing, it's plain rude to other drivers. If we're hearing things, seeing things, Panicking, feeling immense rage – or experiencing any of our personal signals that an attack is coming on – it's time to go home. You can call the folks at your intended destination and tell them you got sick on the road. They will understand.

Or if they don't – are they worth dying for?

If you're too sick even to go home, pull over carefully and take any pill you've got that will help (of course you carry a days' worth of medicine with you everywhere – don't you?). Then crawl into the backseat and wait till you are more functional.

Just a few days ago I was heading home from shopping when I realized I'd forgotten something. I needed a new pot for the tomato plant, which was so overgrown it was dying off. (I am really nuts about my plants. I go into fits of despair if one dies, and think I am an awful person.) This was my last chance at the car for a few days, so I needed to do it *today*. I got back in my car and reached for the ignition, but then I felt the overwhelming confusion and rage in my head. I could barely stand the idea of dealing with my own driveway, much less rush-hour traffic. I felt exhausted at the very idea of unloading the groceries. I tried to convince myself that it was just a *little* errand. It would take only 15 minutes, and then I could rest. It would be easy for anybody else, so why not me?

But I am *not* anybody else. I am me, and I am PASC. I asked myself, "Is a stupid tomato plant worth having a car crash?"

Put like that? No, it wasn't.

I went home. I survived. So did the tomato plant, actually.

These are the kinds of choices we have to make. Pride is not helpful. Throw pride out. It is no use to be a proud dead body. Take the bus instead.

On the other hand, there are times when public transport is not a good idea either. I once got on a bus in the wrong – er – mood. Three blocks later, the bus was at a dead stop, the driver and passengers were yelling, and one person was slightly injured.

Don't ask. It's too stupid to even explain.

They physically restrained me from disembarking until I gave them my name and address. Coincidentally, the address on my ID was obsolete. I tried to tell them that and give them the new one, but they didn't believe me. They thought I was trying to wiggle out of trouble. The bus driver insisted on copying down the old address for the transit authority. So I got off the hook that time – because later on they couldn't find me. Somewhere out there is a random group of people I will *never* be able to apologize to.

We have to decide, sometimes, whether we really can be out in public.

Here's one alternative: most large metropolitan areas have a bus service for the disabled. You can probably qualify if you are honest with them about the extent of your symptoms. Given advance notice, they will pick you up at home and take you straight to your goal, then take you home again at a pre-arranged time. Usually just an application and your doctor's signature are necessary. The drawback is that you have to tell them as much as 24 hours beforehand where you want to go and what time you want to go there.

If you really MUST go out, try to get a friend to walk or drive you. You don't need to go into the gory details. Just say, "I'm feeling very confused. I need some help. Will you go with me?" This is a good choice for psychiatric or therapy appointments, which you should never miss if possible. The professionals can't help you if they can't see you.

Your ace-in-the-hole is to keep a $20 bill stashed somewhere for the odd emergency taxi.

PART FIVE:

All We Can Be

"Our deepest fear is that
we are powerful beyond
measure. It is our light, not
our darkness, that most
frightens us."
- from A Return to Love
by Marianne Williamson

Step Eleven

Communicate With Your Spirit

"Sought through prayer and meditation to improve our conscious contact with our Higher Power as we understood It, praying only for knowledge of Its will for us and the power to carry that out."
--adapted from the Twelve Steps of AA

Step Eleven

If you thought we were done with prayer back in Step Three, think again.

For one thing, surrendering to a Higher Power's guidance and care is something that most of us need to do regularly. We forget.

For another thing the PASC, among all people, really need an integral spiritual life. There are times when it seems we have nothing to cling to. We can't work much; we can't get better; we may be living off the generosity of our relatives or the (limited) tender mercy of the government; maybe we are barely scratching out rent and food in a meager subsidized room in a crummy part of town. And on top of this, things go wrong for us as they do for everyone else. We get sick, we lose friends, our therapists or doctors suddenly retire or move away. Bills come in that aren't covered by Medicare. Program funding changes and leaves us out in the rain. What's going to keep us afloat?

Well, sometimes there isn't anything other than our Higher Power. And that's the time we need the rock-hard sense of belonging and hope provided by a regular spiritual connection. Emergency shouts out to the Universe don't work the same. We need a stable, ongoing relationship with something stronger than we are.

The ideal would be to spend a little time at our spiritual practice each day. Any time of day is appropriate; just some section of time you can get to and remember regularly. You don't even have to be alone, if that's a problem. Your silent thoughts can be directed to the Cosmic at any minute, and it's nobody's business but yours.

We've talked a bit about prayer previously – how to pray, what to say – but I'd like to put in a plug here for extending prayer. It can be more like a meandering conversation than a laundry list of wishes we want filled. It can be a discussion of what's happening in our lives, how we feel about it, where we need help in decision-making. It can be an admission of the things we'd like to be better at, places where we know we're weak. It can be – and I highly recommend this – the place to direct our gratitude list, a nice balance to all those requests and pleas. It feels very different to direct that gratitude to someone rather than just reciting it to ourselves and trying to feel appreciative.

And atop all this, we can pray for the best for the people and causes we care about. But be aware that even here, we must make our requests subject to the Higher Power's will, not our own. There may be some overarching reason why our friends have to go through the things that happen to them; important, life-changing experiences they must have in order to grow.

So be a little humble in your efforts to pray the world better.

Over time, you will find you get results.

Whose Will Be Done?

We do well to remember that in the Universe as a whole it is always the Higher Power's will that prevails, not ours. This is true even if our Higher Power is only our recovery group (or the human race). On a group level, no one person is able to control everything for any significant length of time. Even dictators and military leaders die. We just don't have the leverage to rule the cosmos.

We may, temporarily, get our will done if we fight hard enough or pray hard enough. But if it doesn't go with the flow of what God is doing overall, it will be of little use. If a house is being faced in shingle, and we insist our contribution is three bricks, it's just not going to work very well – for the house or for the bricks.

Mental illness is not part of our conscious will. On the contrary, it is a chilling reminder of how little control we really have. But that does not mean that our lives have to be unsuitable or useless or wasted. We can still be part of the flow of what is beautiful and fitting in this universe. We don't have to stop having wills or wishes or plans. All the Twelve-Step program suggests we do is ask that God take care of those plans, guide them and bring them into fruition in the best possible way.

Then, forget about it.

There is only so much that can be done by foresight, moral awareness, and medical science. The rest falls in the realm of mystery, and strangely enough, life seems to work better this way.

What Else We Can Do

The other great road to oneness with God that the program recommends is meditation. There are many ways to meditate, some formal and some not so formal.

For instance, every time we go out into nature and are struck with wonder at the beauty of it and how it all works together, this is a mini-meditation. Every time we put ourselves totally into an activity we love, and time and self-consciousness just disappear, we have been in a meditative state. When we listen to music and are fully enclosed in its rhythm and beauty, we are meditating. When we sit and quietly seek the truth from ourselves (as in working an inventory) we are also meditating.

My pocket-sized Scribner-Bantam English Dictionary says that to meditate means: 1) to intend, to plan; 2) to ponder, reflect, contemplate.

I have found that even riding a horse can turn into a satisfying meditation of oneness with the horse and its movement. It is the "oneness", the complete attention and love one gives to an activity, that brings such small moments of meditative loveliness into our lives.

We all have opportunities to make these moments for ourselves, sometimes many times a week. Any good sunset can do it.

Formal Meditation

Then there are the formal schools of meditation. This is exercise for the soul.

For the PASC, the goal of meditation is not necessarily "enlightenment" (whatever that is). The goal is to learn to *purposely* alter your consciousness to a beneficial state in which chemical and emotional storms cannot disturb you. Frankly, I can't say I've had a better offer.

The drawback is that, like learning to play the piano, mastery can take years of practice. Luckily, there are short-term benefits as well.

My own meditation habits, at this writing, are very stop-and-go. So I cannot personally assure you of how this works. But meditation has thousands of years of good press. You are unlikely to find any other method of mental healing so well supported or documented.

And it's free. That gives it points over every Western therapy in existence.

Start with 15 minutes; then extend the time as you are able. Meditation, as I understand it (and I am an amateur, remember), involves concentrating on one thing and one only, with complete attention, until your time is up. This may sound easy, but it is actually incredibly hard. The mind wants to spin away in all directions: solve problems, issue warnings, critique the last thing you did, notice the smell of the room. Your job is to keep gently but firmly brushing away these intrusions and going back to looking inward at your chosen focus of concentration. That's it. That's all.

So what is a subject for meditation? Well, it can be something simple, like counting your breaths up till four, or ten, and then starting over again. It can be complex, like visualizing yourself at the bottom of a lake and thinking of a particular subject, and seeing thoughts about this subject rising as bubbles, slowly, one by one. You give each bubble a certain number of seconds of contemplation as it rises to the surface. Then you let it go and pay attention to the next one.

It can be a physical practice, like lying still and feeling the rise and fall of your abdomen, or looking vividly and attentively (without touching) at a seashell. It can be chanting a chosen mantra over and over.

There are many, many ways to meditate, and I do not propose to give an overview here. Somewhere there is one that is right for you. I recommend googling it, or taking a trip to the nearest library. If you are a complete virgin, you might want to try Meditation for Dummies. I also found the book How to Meditate, by Lawrence LeShan, especially helpful, though it's probably out of print now. Any library (remember libraries?) can give you dozens of titles, or DVDs, videos and tapes if you're not into books.

So what is the point of meditation? Why would you want to do it? The official objective is to become closer to a Higher Power, which is exactly what you want out of the Eleventh Step. Most of us would just settle for a little peace of mind. That's a valid goal, too. Meditation is said, with serious practice, to bring an understanding of our oneness with the universe, and show us a whole new view of the world. But even without going so far, there is a lot that it can do for us.

It is credited with all sorts of side benefits, from calming tempers to quitting smoking, losing weight, and promoting general serenity. I don't know the fancy details, but meditating gives us measurably different brain wave patterns. That last is something that is certainly worth working for if you have special chemistry. I don't know about you, but I am not especially fond of the patterns my brain tends to run by itself.

The basic idea is that for the period of meditation, you retreat into a quiet inner place, the core of your self, *the place where you are not sick.* The more often you do this, the easier it will become to be quiet and calm in your daily life even when you are not meditating.

Meditation and prayer are both powerful tools, and you don't need a church to do either. Meditation may be a better alternative for atheists and anyone uncomfortable with religion. Both are free, and they won't hurt you.

Try one. Try both. Try.

Yoga

In my personal experience, the single most powerful type of meditation is physical yoga. This is because it works through your breathing and your body, so it works fast. You *feel* it. You don't need years of practice to achieve inner calm; you'll have some by the end of class.

There are many schools of yoga and numerous ways that people teach it. I can't tell you which one will work best for you. But I will give you some guidelines that I have found helpful.

You want a teacher who is not going to rush you through the various positions. This is not an aerobics class. You will get plenty of work done by going s-l-o-w-l-y, trying to relax into each position as you hold it for a while. The various positions are actually called 'asanas,' or poses. So you should not be rushing from one to the next, but posing, as if for a statue.

You also want to avoid any atmosphere of competition. It makes no difference how 'far' you can go compared to your neighbor. *Any* movement beyond what your body is used to will do you good. You do not have to be beautiful, thin, strong, or flexible. You do not have to have good balance. You don't even have to be able to get completely into the positions. There are often modified postures that are just as useful, if you've got movement restrictions. We have people in my class who've had hip replacements and people who weigh hundreds of pounds, and they do just fine. In fact, they impress the hell out of me.

You just have to be willing to try. A little bit of progress is good enough. You will feel like a new person afterward.

It is extremely important that you breathe fully, in and out deeply, while you are working on this. Any teacher who does not remind you to breathe, or teach you to breathe from your abdomen, is not doing his or her full job. There are lots of good anatomical reasons for this, such as what it does for the circulation and for removing toxins from your blood. But even more important, breathing yogically is *the fastest way to calm your mind.* If all you do is breathe calmly and deeply for an hour, even without the exercises, you will come out in better mental shape than you went in. Add the poses to that breathing, and it's dynamite therapy.

Lastly, I would personally recommend a teacher who does not treat yoga as 'just exercise.' It is an ancient discipline with all kinds of potential for mental, emotional, and spiritual growth, and you will get the most from a teacher who treats it with respect. That doesn't mean they have to be Hindu, or burn incense, or have an idol in the room. But it does mean that they would realize you are there to expand yourself a little, that the way you think is as important as the way you move, and that this is not just a way to sweat off a few calories.

It's also nice to have a period of rest afterward, so that you can enjoy your peacefulness without having to rush back to the rat race. Possibly your teacher will include a time of lying still and resting at the end of the class, and this is ideal. If not, just give yourself five minutes before you hit the highway.

Short of serious psychiatric drugs, I cannot think of *anything* that has helped me more than yoga. I pass this on to you with my whole heart.

Outer Tips for Inner Peace

Strategy 11: Surviving Suicidal Depression

In severe Clinical Depression, you lose all will to live. It's one of the worst things special chemistry can dish out. It's just a chemical shortage, but that's not what it feels like.

The way I've always described it to myself is that the motor has died in me. Everyone has a little, crucial motor that wakes up with them each day and makes them want to go on – at least after a cup of coffee or two. In Clinical Depression, the motor STOPS. It is jammed or broken. Who knows why.

And you don't care. You are perfectly happy to stay in bed all day every day. People don't realize till they've been there that it takes *energy* to give a damn. That's something the people around you, trying frantically to get you 'back to normal,' don't understand.

With time, and maybe the navigation of some crucial life issues, that motor will kick in again. The job of anti-depressants is to jump start it. The danger is that people won't live that long.

In suicidal Depression, you have one job and one only: stay alive until the motor starts. It is gruesome, but possible.

I have been suicidal, I forget how many times. Once I spent 2 whole years in bed. I survived it. This is how.

First and most important: *do not buy into how you feel*. I know it seems like the world is one big kitty-litter box and you are buried at the bottom. *But your brain is lying to you!* That is vitally important to understand. When your thoughts say, "It's not worth living," you can respond, "What a load of crap!"

In rehab they taught us something I never forgot: **Feelings are not facts. Feelings just are**. It's just a broken brain showing you everything through a black filter. It's not real. It's a movie-screen disaster. It cannot kill you all by itself! Only you can do that.

If we have an 'ordinary' Depression and things look dark, we are usually best served by keeping busy and keeping in motion. But if we are flat out suicidal, it just may not be possible. The rules are different when all you can think of is how much you want to die.

Your only job right now is to stay alive, and here are a few tips to help you do that:

1) *Get rid of all weapons.* I have a gun for self-protection (I know that's not very PC). When I start thinking I don't want to live, I give that gun to my therapist and say, "Hold onto this for me for a while." Pills are weapons. If you start thinking of overdosing on your pills, it's time to get somebody to dole them out to you one day at a time. You can do this. Doctors are willing. Your friends would rather do this than see you die.

2) *Get a crisis number and call it any time you have to.* Call your therapist. Ask for extra sessions. Write long letters or journals about how bad you feel. But don't expect your best friends to be able to listen to it every day. They can't even understand, though they may be willing to try. There is no normal person on earth who will be able to stand your current point of view for as long or as often as you will need to vent it. *Use* the professionals. They're there for exactly this.

If there are local prayer lines, you might call them too. A lot of people praying might just make the difference. What could it hurt?

3) *Find something passive to keep yourself occupied.* TV or books or audio tapes or crosswords – *anything* will do if it keeps you from sitting around brooding. Cuddling your cat or stuffed animal helps, too. If you just sit and think, you might crumble. If you have to watch reruns at three in the morning till you finally drift off into a coma, that is better than dying.

This is a good time for that music collection I recommended. This is a good time to take up knitting. This is a good time to play Slinky, or Solitaire, or Marbles. This is a good time to surf endlessly on your computer. Go into a mindless zone where you are just slightly too busy to think about how much you hurt. This is NOT a good time to take up drugs or alcohol. Your lens on the world is already way too distorted as it is.

4) *Keep it simple, and take your medicine.* I know hygiene and moving about socially don't interest you very much right now. I'm going to be different than the textbooks and say that's fine sometimes. If you want to lie dirty in bed all week except when you go get the groceries, OK. Just so you stay alive.

I have a request, though: when you do go for the groceries, take a shower first. It is the kind thing to do, and it will make you feel marginally better. Also, get up for therapy and to pick up your prescriptions, even if you don't get out of bed for anything else.

NEVER neglect your pills. *Especially now.*

5) *Handling family*: If you have children, this is more complicated. You might have to develop a routine of minimum chores to do each day before you go back to bed. Show your spouse this section of the book, and tell him/her to bring in help. S/he's lucky to have a partner at all right now. Normal services have been interrupted! Business as usual is just not on the menu, most days. Make sure your children understand that you love them, but you are very sick and need to rest a lot.

6) *If you're employed*: If you are employed, it's very difficult. Of course you have to shower and get up. Maybe you're not sure you can keep that going. You might consider a leave of absence – especially if your performance is so bad you're close to getting fired anyway. That happened to me once, and I had to beg for another chance and go on probation.

It is very hard to do a good job when all you can think of is that you wish you weren't breathing any more. If you can get on welfare or disability to tide you over, now is the time to do it. Public-income programs exist for the times when you can't support yourself.

7) *Do try to eat somewhat decently.* Don't survive on Twinkies and Cokes. I've done that, and it sucks. When you get out of bed at last and find you've gained 40 pounds, you're going to be pissed.

Tip: when you do get around to losing the weight, you will probably need to take in 300 calories less than a person without medications. So the average 1500-calorie-a-day 'diet' intake (for most females) comes down to 1200. That's not much. It's rough sticking to that strict a regimen. Better not to gain it in the first place.

8) *This is not the time to make major life decisions*. They will for sure be all wrong. Especially do not get married.

9) For suicidal thoughts, here are some counter-thoughts that helped stop me at the worst times, the times I was actually making plans to die:

--Think of the mess and ugliness. What will it be like for the person who finds your body? Do you want to make a friend shovel your brains off the floor? That happened to someone I know.

--Think about FAILING at suicide and having to live with the consequences. There was once, they say, a boy in my community who shot himself in the mouth, cop-style. Somehow, he missed the most vital parts and stayed alive. However, he became a quadriplegic, and will now have to be cared for all his life by his family. AND HE STILL HAS TO LIVE WITH ALL THOSE AWFUL THOUGHTS IN HIS HEAD. But now he can't even talk about them to anyone.

Wouldn't you rather check into a hospital than have this happen to you?

-Think about what comes **after**. Oh, I know what you want from death. You want OBLIVION. You want it all to be OVER. But is that really what happens at death? Do you know? Does anyone? I'm not going to try to scare you with hellfire, but consider this: what if they just send you straight back to earth to do it again? What if this is a test, and the protocol for failing is even worse?

Maybe the only way out is through. 'Rest' and 'silence' may not be on the menu at all.

--If you really can't control yourself, the hospital is where you belong.

-10) The real and final reason for living through this: *Everything changes.* Your brain is telling you that this horribleness is the way it will be, forever and ever, amen. But your brain is *wrong*.

I wanted to die, for the first time, when I was 19. I was poor and out of my mind and was scrounging the gutters for dropped change to buy food with – when I wasn't shoplifting. I had dropped out of college, I had no skills, and I could see no future. But I went to say a last goodbye to a friend, and she talked me out of it. Thank God for her, because I was dead serious.

It wasn't the last time I wanted to die. There were to be many others. As I mentioned, I spent two years pretty much without leaving bed in my late twenties. Each time I was suicidal felt just as bad as the last time, and each time I felt I had no future.

Today, I have a four-bedroom house in a pricey suburb, I'm going to college again, and I'm living with the love of my life – who happens to be a lot more fun than I even dreamed he would be. My pills and my preventive measures have made my symptoms nearly invisible, if I'm careful. I get to write every day if I want to. I am so happy, old friends tell me I glow. But I had to stay alive long enough to get here.

What if I had missed all this?

There was no way to see from there to here. There was no evidence that it would turn out this way, or any good way at all. Life is not a straight line. It takes all kinds of turns and you *do not know* what is in your future, no matter how it looks from right here.

Stick around for what comes next. I guarantee it won't stay the same.

Don't be another statistic. We don't need more statistics. We need more people like you.

Step Twelve

Share What You Learn

"Having had a spiritual awakening as a result of these steps, we tried to carry this message to the mentally ill, and to practice these principles in all our affairs."
--adapted from the Twelve Steps of AA

Step Twelve

When we wake up we open our eyes. That's what we did in the First Step: opened our eyes to our true condition, and admitted that we did not have a solution. Next, having opened our eyes, what do we see?

One of the signs of spiritual awakening is our realization that we are not alone. We are seen, known, and loved by a Power greater than ourselves. We need not feel abandoned in our difficult condition; we can look for help beyond our personal resources.

What follows is a life lived in a larger context. If we are not alone in an empty universe – if we are noticed and loved and unique – then *what we do matters*. Ethics become an integral part of our everyday life. We can no longer be happy doing something shoddy or cruel and saying, "Who cares?" or "Who will know?" We become aware that our acts never go unseen, and that they have consequences. We become morally aware beings.

This is not to say that we become stuffy, righteous, pompous, or perfect. It simply means that we give some thought to what we do. Our personal standards of what is best <u>may</u> be part of an accepted body of beliefs; but they can just as easily be internal, personal standards. It is not always as simple (or as complex) as those of a church or society.

Our goals in life may change. We might still want that car or house or girlfriend, but we know now that this is not all there is to want. Some of our goals will be about growth and self-improvement regardless of whether we get social approval out of that. Some of our goals will be beyond the personal, more than just about ourselves or our lifetimes. We become aware of where we stand in the long line of the millions of mentally ill people throughout the ages. We become concerned, beyond our own survival, with the welfare of the ill and psychotic around us. Feeling compassion and acceptance for ourselves, we feel it for them also.

No longer blaming ourselves and shaming ourselves for our condition, we do not need to wade in self-pity or excuses. We deal squarely with what we have done, and we forgive ourselves for what we can't improve. We become more forgiving.

More than anything else, we learn to value simple things that others take for granted. A clear mind. A good mood. A peaceful hour.

These are gradual things. I do not say that we become saints overnight, or poster children for the PASC community. But we come to feel an inner strength that informs all we do. We are not bitter. We are not regretful or angry. We no longer measure ourselves by the usual ladder of outward achievements, but by our own internal vision of what we can reasonably do and be.

It becomes natural, then, to notice when others are suffering the way we did, and help them out if we are in any position to do so. Often, there may be nothing we can materially do. But we can tell them, 'Hey, me too.' We can show them they are not guilty and not alone. We can share whatever we know that is helpful, including the Twelve Steps for peace of mind: maybe we'll enter an ongoing discussion on the Web, or subscribe to a newsletter that helps support and inform the PASC community. Maybe we'll volunteer some time at an organization for others like us, even if all we can commit to is licking stamps once in a while. Maybe we just make a point of visiting our friends who are still hospitalized.

Whatever else we do, we accept each day as it comes, try to be flexible in dealing with it, and look for the gift or the lesson concealed behind our pain. We keep the Steps as part of the pattern of our fractured lives, and meditate or pray or do yoga regularly. Do our best and then let go of the outcome, leaving results to whatever Power we believe in. Admit our faults, try to mend any harm we do, and try to rise to a higher vision of what kind of person we can be <u>in the hours when we get to choose.</u> The reward is more peace and balance. We are worthy. And we can contribute to the beauty and shape and hope of the world, just by not giving up.

We cannot change our ultimate condition, but we can start to change society's view of it. Mental illness does not occur in a vacuum. Those who are able to function have an obligation to befriend those who cannot; to help and protect them where possible; to show them compassion; to help relieve the unfair feelings of shame. It is our duty to explain them to the world, when they cannot explain themselves.

And there is a mission to the worldwide community. We are only now emerging from centuries of fear and isolation and imprisonment and stigma. Those of us who can live somewhat normal lives have a responsibility to produce and contribute what we can. We also have a mandate to fight stigma by disclosing who we are and demonstrating every day to the world at large that the PASC *can* produce and contribute. Just by holding a rational conversation and not being scary, you are contributing to the reputation of all PASC people everywhere.

There is more to be done with us than warehouse us and sedate us. There is more that we can offer the world than fear and bewilderment. We are the only ones who can do it. No one else really knows what it's like.

We can't supply the money. We can't cure ourselves. But we alone can give the world some reasons they should care.

Some Thoughts on the Mental Health System

I asked everyone I interviewed this question: If you could change one thing in the mental health system, what would it be? Here are their answers:

Lisa:

> "Financially, I'm very lucky...I'm aware, however, that many are not so fortunate. This is unfair beyond measure...Without insurance I couldn't afford my medications, and there is no way these pills are worth what they're charging. I hope something can be done about the

pharmaceutical companies robbing us blind in the near future."

Shelley:

"Availability of many, many places. Like, it wouldn't be so *hard* to find a psychiatrist or psychologist! You have to go to this guy, [and then] this guy, [and then] this guy, [and then] this guy... They're all, they'd be, like, at the *corner store*, or at Walgreen's. You'd go up to the pharmacy and say, 'You know, I'm Bipolar, and I need a doctor,' and they'd say, 'Oh, here's one in this neighborhood.' There'd be, like, neighborhood based facilities. It'd be so much easier to find mental health care. Like the 7-11. Go out, get some milk. Whatever."

Eddie has a similar view:

"It would be easy in and easy out, with the formal insurance system – most people, you gotta go to only your HMO, and they're X number of miles away, and they're not ready to see you just yet, AND they want you to see your general physician first – or you even should see him first, because he's kind of the central information hub? If he's out of the loop really bad mistakes could be made. So there needs to be one computerized thing; they type everything that you say there. When another doctor pulls it up it comes up right on his screen: everything about you. That's really good.

"What I would do, is I would have a really easy entry system. So when a person's undergoing an Anxiety Disorder, there's a 24-hour place where they can go to and start working on it right away. See a psychiatrist right away. Get medicine right away. Or you could come in to the emergency room right now, see a doctor right now, and get a prescription right now. But it would cost you $4,000 for ten minutes. (Laughter) OK, that's scarier than the disease, practically.

"So right now it's a punitive thing. If you're becoming mentally ill, you're going to have to do a ton of work...

"Either way, you're kind of guilty in the sense that you're in trouble. And we're going to make sure that you are super-discouraged. So we're going to design it so getting QUICK help, there'll be big penalties for you. So that's the thing I would change: to make psychiatric emergencies to get immediate and really local access to help.

"Like, this hospital here has a fully blown mental hospital. But they'll charge you, like, $350 for a ten-minute visit. So...and then they'll say, 'As a medical doctor I could give you some psychiatric meds – if it's an emergency. But this really needs to be monitored by a psychiatrist. We have one, but that'll be another $150 intake, plus she doesn't have anything open for a week and a half. And, sorry that you'll be sort of Panicking between then.'

"Yeah. Good luck, I say."

According to Nelson, the same problem pertains in Britain:

"In the UK...it would be nice to HAVE a mental care system!

"That may seem a little unfair – at least I am getting help. However, if I had not been deemed an 'emergency' case by my MD I'd not have been seen by a Consultant Psychiatrist for about 3-4 months. And I've already been waiting to see a Psychotherapist for 17 months ...Mental Health and Geriatrics are at the bottom of the Government's priorities."

Gabriel's comment was:

"One thing I would change about the American mental health system would be to have psychiatrists on staff in family practice clinics, instead of off in their own little psych practices. I think that would alleviate some of the stigma associated with mental illness."

Lisa, the mom from Alabama, also feels we need more coordinated efforts:

"Before pills are dosed out, a person should have a complete medical exam to rule out hormonal problems and other physical conditions which can mimic the symptoms of mental illness. Hypnosis can profoundly assist one in coping with daily obstacles, obsessions, compulsions, etc...I feel strongly that professionals need to work together...this should be included in the analysis...If they are truly professionals, it's their job to give us a professional diagnosis and treatment."

Some people would argue that having a 'case manager' takes care of this problem. Perhaps. But in 30 years of treatment and more than five hospitalizations, no one has ever suggested assigning a case manager to me. So I suspect this is an under-used option.

Pablo feels we need to watch the definitions we use for mental illness:

> "You get into a pretty tricky game of words. Because what is – quote unquote – a mental illness? Some of the things I have read lately, the professional attitude is changing. Let's digress for a moment.

> "Back in the sixties it was thought that people who were gay – it was a mental illness! It was right there in the book!

> "And they changed that. Now there's even such a belief that people who have my type of condition or even Depression, they say, it is *not* a mental illness! You can call it a *condition*, but it's not a mental illness. Real division there, in what we can call a mental illness. This is the problem in language. Because in language, we tend just to lump everything together.

> "Oh. You're a little goofy here or you walk down the street with no clothes on, oh, you must be mentally ill. And there's all kind[s] of other [reasons], maybe you just want to act out or whatever. And that's all in the eye of the beholder."

Only Sally said that she would leave the system alone:

"I used to think I would change a lot.
But now that I'm on the spiritual path, I would
say, not much."

Sally believes that anything one encounters – anything –
is karmic and meant to teach us. In my opinion, there's a lot
going for approaching life in this way, whether it's true or not.
Even if a hardship is not 'meant' to teach me, I'd rather learn
something than just go through all that pain for nothing.

Jessica, the graduate student with generalized Anxiety
Disorder, Depression and ADHD, says we need an attitudinal
shift.

"Trying to see people as human beings
rather than just a conglomeration or a bunch of
symptoms. Try to deal with people as people.
Don't just sit around among yourselves talking
about, 'Well, how are we going to deal with
The Borderline? The Borderline does this and
that.' Stop relying so much on the stupid
diagnosis and start relying on actually having
conversations with the people and seeing them
as people instead of an underserved group of
this or that.

"Yeah. A need for more humanity and
more real focused help instead of, 'Oh, you're
down there, I'm up here, I can help you' type
of thing."

What would you change? Come to think of it, why aren't
you trying to change it right now? You'd be astounded how
many groups exist in our favor. Check out the nationally based
organizations in the 'Resources' section in the back of this
book. Even if you're not in any shape to be politically active,
your dues help contribute to the special chemistry community
and its causes. Or just keep informed and vote when it concerns
the PASC.

As I write this, everything has just changed forever in the American health system. The Health Care Reform bill was signed into law by President Obama on March 19, 2010. When all the improvements have been phased in, some of the recurrent problems the PASC have faced will be over. We will no longer be refused insurance just because we are PASC (the notorious 'pre-existing condition' clause). And though they can put annual caps on how much they will cover, insurance companies will no longer be able to say, "OK, you've been in the psychiatric wing too many times in your lifetime – we won't cover that any more." There are no lifetime caps. And for those of us who are on Medicare, the 'donut hole' limits on prescription spending will eventually be eliminated. We won't be liable, after our initial $2,700, for up to $4,000 in prescription expenses before the government starts chipping in again. This is important, because many psychiatric drugs are extremely expensive – especially the newest ones, the breakthrough discoveries, the ones without generic equivalents yet. Our medication needs can easily run into the high thousands every year.

However, the basic question of mental health parity remains unresolved. Typically, insurers cover lots of physical care and very little psychiatric care. It remains to be seen whether costs for psychiatric care will come down in the wake of reform, or whether availability of service will be affected.

Best Advice

When I interviewed other special chemistry folks for this book, I asked each this question: If you could give just one piece of advice to the mentally ill everywhere, what would it be? Some of these answers have already been given in the text.

Shanna:

> "Don't hold it in to the extent that you're going to explode. Just hold it in long enough to talk to somebody."

Vivien:

"Have hope that things can change, that life is worth living, and don't commit suicide. Because we don't know, things could change."

Lisa:

"My advice to the mentally ill population is to insist on an accurate diagnosis. If what is being done doesn't feel right, it probably isn't. It's okay to want to feel better, there's nothing at all selfish about that. You may have forgotten what it feels like to feel normal, or you may have never known, but your intuition knows."

Jessica says to trust ourselves:

"Take what other people give you – those who do not have mental illness, a doctor or whoever – take what they say with a grain of salt. Because they don't really know. You've got to trust yourself more, because there's a lot of stigma in this society and there's a lot of fear around people being different. Learn to really keep your own counsel on things, and maybe network with other people who have mental illness. It's just kind of the reality we live in."

Nelson:

"You know how some people catch a nasty flu? Well that's all this is – it's not your fault, it's an illness and, in time, you WILL feel better."

Gabriel:

> "I'm not about to go on about hitting bottom or looking on a bright side. I simply believe that life is worth living...take concrete steps toward a goal...keep [your] feet on the ground. That's important. I've learned that ignoring a problem doesn't make it go away."

Eddie says,

> "Don't have any ego about having multiple layers of backup plans. Know what the big charities are in your area. Know what the government programs are and where they're located. Have a backup plan of where you would live if you can't live where you're living now. In every area, be prepared.

> "Throughout your life there'll be multiple downward spirals...never stop looking at plans. Never stop saying, 'What is my backup plan now?'"

Sally:

> "In other cultures your 'illness' would be seen as a gift. It's all about perspective. You can choose how you see your situation. I would give this advice to anyone at all...the water glass stops at the middle. It is always in your power to see the glass as half full or half empty."

Outer Tips to Inner Peace

Strategy 12: Surfing the System

I have a reputation among my friends for getting the most out of the bureaucracy. Here are some tips gleaned from 20+ years in the mental health system.

First of all, **don't expect fast results**. If you need housing next week, start counting up friends' sofa-beds right now. Approaching the red-tape establishment in desperation puts you at a nasty disadvantage. Public employees often don't listen well to the urgent or the stressed. They get very huffy about the pace at which they will move.

Expect that big benefits, like Disability, will take up to two years to achieve. Small ones, like assistance paying for your pet's vaccinations, about six weeks. Government-sponsored benefits are always harder to get. There are more hoops to jump through. Volunteer groups have been formed strictly to help you. Government employees have been trained to safeguard the taxpayers' money and keep out frauds – so, sadly, you are considered a fraud till proven otherwise.

So that's the first rule: give it time.

The second is: **never miss deadlines or appointments**. Even if you are sick, or need an attendant, manage it or reschedule it. If you miss, you can mess up the whole works and they can deny your application on the grounds that you 'didn't do your part.'

The other tips follow in no particular order.

Get everything in writing – and keep the paperwork. If it's an interview or a phone call, be sure to write down any instructions or promises made, along with the date and who told you.

Keep names and phone numbers you find helpful. If you find an employee with a surprisingly good attitude or good information, ask for that person by name next time you call that office. You may even want to call them again about more general info, or a referral. "Hi, Michael. It's Deborah again. I just wanted to ask you: what department do I call for X situation? Do you have any numbers there?" Contacts are priceless, and might even become friends over the years. But don't wear out your welcome.

Keep copies of everything YOU send. It is a savvy trick to send things by certified and/or registered mail, so you can *prove* an office got something on such-and-such a date. If the office completely loses the information you spent six weeks gathering, and you have no copies, you are S.O.L. It does happen. Horrifying but true. So be persnickety about this.

Get friendly with your phone book. When you need something and don't know where to start, look in the city, county, and federal pages at the front. Think of other names for it if you can't find it at once. It may be under 'Human Resources' instead of 'Social Services.' The Internet is great, but not all of us have it, or are good with it. The phone book is free.

Go in person if you can. If you want a service and you can get to the office, get presentable and go there. A friend of mine needed housing. We went together to the county office and received a 25-page handout of places to look and agencies to contact! Nobody's going to give you that over the phone. You have to be there. And the human touch works wonders.

Be concise and polite. Losing your temper will get you thrown out the door, hung up on, or given the worst possible service. If you do lose it, take a deep breath, then smile and say sincerely, "I'm sorry. This is a stressful process and sometimes I get angry." Even though these people are dealing with the mentally ill all the time, they have few people skills and no psychological skills or patience (my apologies to the few shining exceptions!). DO NOT TAKE IT PERSONALLY. Paranoia will end the conversation every time, and get you marked down as a troublemaker. Their attitude is NOT about you.

Do not tell a long, detailed sob story. Do not try to make them feel sorry for you or give them every last detail. They've heard it all. They don't care.

Have plenty of proof of your claims. Back up your diagnosis, your work history, your hospitalizations, and anything else they'll question. Get paperwork from doctors and employers, or their agreement to back you up if someone calls them. Have a lease to prove your residence, or a friend who will verify that you are staying with them.

In bureaucracies, paperwork is God. You cannot afford to be disorganized about this.

Getting Organized: What if you are disorganized by nature?

Here's a simple system.

1) Get a box. Not a huge box, just one about the size of a milk crate or a standard box of books.

2) Get some folders – one for each agency you're trying to get help from. Write the name of each agency on a folder – Medicare, SSI, Disability, Housing, Medicare Part D, Therapist, Psychiatrist….whatever the issues are you're working on.

3) Every time you get a piece of paper about that issue, put it in the right folder *on top* of whatever's there.

4) Every time you send out something to that agency, put a copy of it *on top* of whatever's there.

5) Every time you have a phone call or make notes or memos, or do ANYTHING about that issue or agency, you write it down and put it in the right folder *on top*.

6) DO NOT THROW AWAY ANY OF THE PAPERS.

This system keeps it simple. Whatever is most recent is right on top. Whatever is going on will be right there when you reach for it. Even if it's old and somebody starts making a fuss about it, you know it's just further down in the stack.

So all you have to do is develop a habit of putting each paper *in the folder the second you put it down*. Don't put them anywhere else. Don't leave them somewhere 'temporarily' or 'till I can get to it.' If you use this system your papers will always be in the same place every time, and nothing will be missing.

It doesn't matter if the notes are crumpled or scribbled or have phone numbers scrawled on them in 3 colors of ink, or coffee spilled on them. It doesn't have to be neat. It just has to be COMPLETE and FINDABLE. Just keep the box in the same old corner of the closet, or whatever.

The rest of your life can be as messy as you want.

Phrases to use when you hit a wall: "What is your name?" (write it down, in front of them. People act differently when they know they will be held responsible.) "Is there *someone else I can talk to*?" "Can I speak with your *supervisor*?" (If the supervisor/manager/boss is out, ask ,"When can I reach him/her, then?") Or, try calling another day, and speak to someone else. Not everybody has the same information – or the same chip on their shoulders.

If you are completely stuck? Memorize this one: "If you were in my shoes, where would you look next?" *And then get the number.* Inside numbers are often much more efficient than the general numbers, especially if they give you a specific person or department. Another reason to *always write numbers down.*

Always follow the rules. Read the fine print. Do not lie. If you play by their rules, they can't throw you out.

It took me two years to get Disability. On appeal, they were going to say 'no' again because I had earned more money than their maximum in only one month out of the entire previous year. I studied the figures and saw that the month in question was a month with five weeks – and thus had one extra paycheck! I was *not* earning more per hour or more per month. It was just a longer month.

When I pointed that out to the investigator, I won my case.

Use reason. Use their own rules against them. Use the system's loopholes. Read the fine print. There are such things as public-assistance lawyers to help you with this. Find one if you need one.

It can be OK sometimes to leave something immaterial out of your answers. I once had my doctor look over a Disability Review form, and he said I should cross out the information that I took long walks every day. He said in their minds, if I could exercise, I wasn't very sick. Ludicrous, but true. So I left that sentence out. It didn't change the basic facts of my condition.

Having a doctor or experienced friend look your stuff over, if you can, is a good idea.

But don't outright lie. If you get caught, the game is over. You have just made things harder for the next person in line, too.

Being in trouble does NOT excuse you from ethics.

Follow through to the bitter end. If they say 'no,' but there is an appeal process, then appeal! Some agencies routinely say 'no' just to weed people out. They may give you bogus reasons such as, "You can walk and follow instructions. Therefore you are employable." (True story. Happened to a friend of mine, completely incapable of supporting himself for the last few decades.) Get a doctor on your side, and go for the second round. If there are community-service lawyers in your area, get one.

Do not call or show up while upset or symptomatic. Reschedule. This one is self-explanatory. The only exception is if you are in the throes of trying to prove how sick you are. In that case, a picture is worth a thousand words. But bring someone to interpret you.

Never give up.

I know this sounds like a lot, but think about it this way: How much is a free income and medical care, *for life*, worth to you? If someone said, "Look, the deal is, you have to work for us for two years, and it will be a really nutty two years, but after that you'll never have to work again; we'll just feed you, give you money"...would you do it? Hmmm?

Don't be ashamed, and don't have false pride. The American public, as a majority, over numerous decades, has decided that some people need to be helped, and is willing to pay for some of it. You are entitled to these services, if you can prove your case.

And *keep your ears open*. There are all kinds of services out there which are never advertised. For instance, if you were wondering how to afford the yoga class I recommended, go the YMCA and ask, and you will find that they offer scholarships for low-income people. Or, for instance, some charities help with deposit fees on apartments if all you have is one month's rent. Some cities have groups that will actually pay for your pet care, or offer you help cleaning your apartment. The gas and electric company once paid my entire several-hundred-dollar heating bill, the worst bill of the winter, on proof of low income and my promise not to re-apply for a year. (This service was called REACH. I don't know if it still exists.) There are telephone discounts, public-transportation discounts, and free mammograms for low-income patients, in some areas.

The point is, you have to stop being proud and ASK. Say, "I have a disability and a low income. Are there any special programs to help me out?"

Trade info like this with friends, and listen to any services they know about – make a note even if you don't need it now. You may someday. I keep a file called Community Resources full of these snippets and leads. They've saved me and my friends over the years.

You can do this. I did. Just keep good records and be very, very patient.

If you can't do it, find someone who cares enough, show them this section, and ask for help.

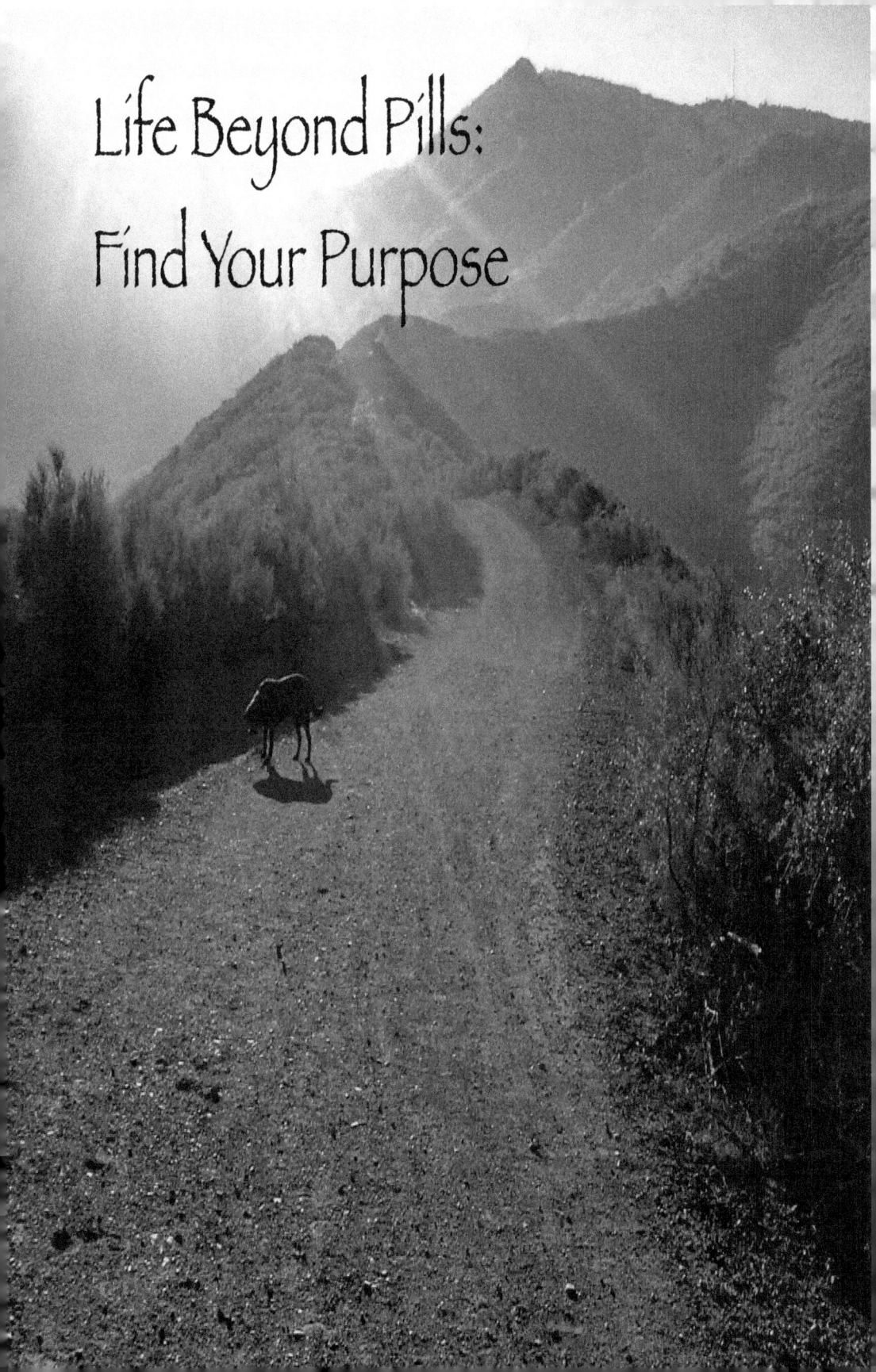

Life Beyond Pills:

Find Your Purpose

Life Beyond Pills: Find Your Purpose

Beyond achieving as much sanity as possible, everybody needs a purpose in life. Once you have some grip on your symptoms, it's time to start thinking of goals again. It may be a more slippery grip than you had hoped for, but at some point you must stop aiming for perfection and get on with the show. And do remember that we live in fortunate times, when more effective medicines are being discovered every year. If you have a symptom that doesn't respond to any known medicine, maybe it will respond to next year's new find.

Understand that your symptoms may never be 'handled.' Even medicine that works now may not work forever.

For instance Nelson, my English interviewee, was direct as ever about his results so far:

> "[I'm] pissed off that my progress is so slow! It seems I have four steps forward and three back. Just as I start feeling strong in myself again, more like the ole 'me,' I slip down into a low and become weepy, often for little or no good reason at all. It's okay being weepy on my own, but not so good when it's in company!"

Shanna, even at her young age, has already dealt with the on-and-off results we sometimes get from our medicines.

> "Every medicine that I've been on, I get immune to it. So, Abilify, I'm starting to get immune to it. It's not working any more. And the only thing that does work, it makes me eat. I eat and eat and eat."

You cannot wait 'till things get better' forever. Whatever shape you are in, you still have a life to live.

Ultimately, special chemistry is not the only determining factor in your life. It is just one of many. As Shanna said, "If I don't make it too big of a deal, it won't be...and you know, a lot of people can come out of this."

What do you personally do to make your life worthwhile? Lisa replies this way:

> "I look within myself and analyze my conscience to bring quality and purpose to my life. Everyone needs hopes, dreams, something to look forward to. I ask myself often: 'What is truly important to you, what really makes you happy?' The answers are various. We also need something that is uniquely our own, some thing we accomplish and can be proud of. Even on the worst days I remind myself that I have value."

Of course, you'll have certain constraints. If your original goal was to be fabulously rich, or become a powerful politician, these roads may now be closed to you at least for the time being.

Nelson says it most succinctly:

> "How do [I] cope financially? Not well since I lost my job largely due to this illness. Keeping my expenses in control isn't quite as easy as it is meeting my wife's expectations! I lost 2/3rds of my income as I fell from a salary to a pension."

It's time to sift and hone down that dream. What did you want *out* of being rich? Was it really all the things you could buy? Or was it just being 'happy'? What did that happiness really consist of? Was it a feeling of safety, or freedom, or abundance? There are other ways to achieve these feelings. Was it all the good you could do for the world? You can still do lots of good on a smaller scale.

Money is the sticking point in PASC life goals. Most of us cannot work full-time – some not even part-time.

May I suggest that you are being given, instead, something absolutely priceless? Time.

In the end time is what people want the most, and cannot bargain for. David Crosby once sang a very beautiful song about death that began, "Time is the final currency. Not money. Not power."

Anybody who has ever pleaded with death for just a few more months with a loved one can tell you how precious time is. Nothing replaces it.

If you cannot work, you have time to think. Time to get to know yourself, to visit friends, to skip the rush hour and tend your window garden instead. You can sit in a sidewalk café and relax while other people rush anxiously by on their way to some crucial appointment. Do you know how much some people would give for just what you have?

Granted, you get this gift of time because you have to spend some of it being pretty damn sick. But when you are functional, you have sheets and billows of time. Use it wisely. Use it to figure out how to get some alternate version of your dream.

I am not saying your life must have an upward trajectory of achievement. You are beyond that now: there are no ladders to climb in the nuthouse. But each of us needs something fulfilling and satisfying to do.

Sally had the most to say on the topic of making a fulfilling life. She starts out this way:

> "Well, [special chemistry] can be seen as a whammy, not a good thing. You know. But actually you could use it to your advantage, you know. I have all this extra time because I am 'not supposed to work.'

> "I've been on SSI since I was eighteen

and unable to work because of it. At first, it was a blessing even with half a school load to not have to work. It took me six years to get through junior college, including the delay of a breakdown. When I reached four years and had to go full time, it was still a blessing. I was studying psychology. I had to study a lot. Now I am finishing my BA career with my true calling, art. I have more time now, not constantly doing homework.

"All the time to think because I don't work was overwhelming to manage at first. These days I find myself sitting and processing countless issues for more than one hour sometimes. It has become a blessing."

Everybody needs a dream – even just a little one. Without a purpose, life turns into a series of days staring at the wall. Without a purpose, you're just waiting for it to be over. And you will find all kinds of ways to destroy yourself. Some are even legal.

Shelley speaks of using alcohol while facing a serious case of Hepatitis C:

"I was drinking to die. I was, totally…if I drink I will die, in the next, say, 24 months. If I start drinking heavily now. If I want to die – If I'm in the mood to die, just go back to vodka again. It's easy."

Life without a dream is the most pernicious form of suicide.

The primary problem the PASC have with jobs is consistency. Maybe they can function OK one day, but not the next. Maybe they could work for five hours, but not for eight. You can do some amazing things, but not forever. Maybe you'll be fine for months but one day you come to work delusional. High-pressure stuff is out.

Pablo muses on the working world:

> "...the only job I ever enjoyed was the first job I had, which was being a newspaper boy. I liked it. Because I was my own boss. You did your own collecting of money. You kept your own books. You were a small business person. And it was great!

> "Then I found out that that's not the way the real world works, when it comes to employment. You know, the traditional idea of a boss yelling at you that you did something wrong all the time.

> "The one thing I did like about [warehousing] is I had no contact with the public. Only once did I have [a position] where you have to act like a salesperson. Because that can be so – people can be off the wall with their demands.

> "...You know I often mused to myself that if I had the brains I would have loved to be a research scientist, sitting in some lab all day long; and then you go to your own home at night and do your thing; you still have your social contact, you know, you're not a complete isolate.

> "...the real world can be very devastating to those who have – those who are easily agitated.

"And for someone like me – you see, if you think you've always got to try to compete and compete and compete and compete and you can't do it or you never get ahead, it becomes such a laborious and defeating way to live. And it gets – I've never been that kind of person.

"...I think the rat race is very bad for all of us who have those problems.

"...usually, people who have some kind of mental illness are a lot better off without that kind of pressure. "

Shelley Scirocco managed to work as a special education teacher for three years, using her intuitive understanding of the mentally damaged:

"Oh, yeah! I made a *great* living up in Seattle! Years ago...For, like, three whole years. I wanted to see if I could do it. And I became this special ed, you know, teacher, and I was, like, very conservative, straight, and I played the game. Well, I – I used my Manic Depression to play that game. 'Oh, yes, I've heard about that. Oh, yes, the theory I've been reading about lately is dadadadada...' I just, like, researched some shit and people loved me. I was very – they thought I was just a genius. And I was *excellent*. Kids LOVED me! It was insane! I was, like, *such* a good employee! But that was when I still had energy – I was making really good money...unbelievable. I *loved* that life.

"But then I got real sick...and everything changed."

But let's say you really can't work at all. Maybe all you can think of these days is, "I am poor. My career is ruined. My girlfriend is gone."

Let me suggest that you have escaped a giant trap.

How many people, in their heart of hearts, really want to spend their life in the service of someone else for 65 years, never doing anything new or special for themselves? How many people want a partner who is not going to stick by them when things get tough, who is only there for the goodies and the fun times? There's a reason they call it 'the rat race.' Did you really want nothing more than to be a rat?

Nelson describes his change of heart:

> "The brief brush with Oblivion causes one to take a fresh perspective on Life...One thing that has come out of it is that I no longer wish to be driven by myself or anyone else (take heed, wife!) to earn money for its own sake. In other words, I wish to have employment that I feel is worthy, good, altruistic and ethical."

This is your ideal chance to make something unique of your life. To become a consultant or freelancer or inventor or artist or expert home tailor, or just to whittle tiny statues of wolves or goddesses. Anything you love and do well could lead to an occupation which you do *on your own terms*.

Sally told me some of her parameters for involvement in activities and work:

> "It's all done in your own creation, your creation of your own schedule. Because there's two things – I'm naturally not a day person, and I naturally have a problem with people telling me what to do – I'm a sweetheart! People love me! But I have a

problem with authority. I'd rather tell myself what to do."

If you don't have any skills you want to use, this is a great time to go back to school. With Disabled Student Centers and Equal Opportunity Programs, a small community college class almost pays for itself. And you can take it as slowly as you need to: one class at a time, if necessary (that's what I'm doing). Go to whatever disability program your college offers; have your doctor back you up; and get the special concessions that will make it all possible for you.

Because you are free now. There's no one to impress any more. You're not competing with the mainstream. You are free to be an absolutely unique individual.

Pablo sees it this way:

> "... getting involved in things that gave me satisfaction.

> "Doing photography. Writing poetry. Getting out to those particular activities that really appeal. The things that appeal to me today started in – even when I was preteen. Hiking. Camping. Bicycling. Photography. Poetry. Theatre work and so forth.

> "...those things which hold so much interest, give you so much pleasure and enjoyment. And you need to do them every single day.

> "People-watch, read the news. What I remember from my high school sociology as 'you're in the aggregate.' You're not interacting with other people in any way, but it just makes you feel good, particularly if you're around people who you think are like you are, you

know. You may not know that for a fact, but you perceive that. So you're in the aggregate setting, it makes you feel good. Yeah, so [you have] the coffee, and you can daydream a little. I've had some actual experiences where I was in some coffee houses in Paris. And that's a long time ago, but I can think, 'Ah, I'm back in Paris again.' You know. It's a little fantasy trip, but it makes you feel good. So you can do that.

"You can do these things that keep you feeling good, connected...because the flip side is Depression."

And don't give up on money completely. Networking, not cash, is the secret to success. If you get known for what you do well, opportunities could follow.

Sally sees her future as both an artist and a spiritual counselor. She looks at her alternatives this way:

"I don't think you can really separate the artist thing and the [special chemistry] thing. I think in a way it comes as a package, at least for me. So, whatever you want to call it, I don't really fit in with society's norms and rules...I don't want to play those games.

"But to make the money, you have to play those games. So I realize that there is a way for me, which is something I like about America: there is sort of a way for everyone. To play the game. So I have a feeling I'm going to be in business for myself."

What about a home-based business? Your room is as good as any place to begin. You might start with a windowsill herb garden and end up the as the city's chief supplier of saffron. Saffron is worth its weight in gold in some parts of the world, did you know that? Many people with large incomes started by creating their own unique niche in their local economy.

I look at it this way: if I had never been stopped by my disease, the rat race would have eaten me. I was in international banking, believe it or not. I was good at what I did, reconciliations and investigations and bookkeeping. I could have continued working with my nose in a pile of papers the rest of my life, scraping a living, probably never making very much. *I might never have found my way to writing.* I would have ignored my strongest dream in favor of the security of a regular paycheck and a life of quiet desperation. And I would have stayed alcoholic, too, because ignoring my dream was killing me inside, and I had to drink to drown that pain.

You don't have to be 'normal' to make a difference in the world. Join a mental health organization. Write a few letters on mental health issues. Or just go to meetings and tell people there is hope. There is life beyond the pill bottle.

Think in terms of modifying your old goals. If you wanted to work with children, and people won't let you anymore, why not invent a new toy or game for them? Or how about studying human development and coming up with an advanced new preschool curriculum that will knock the socks off the establishment? You're the one who has the time to think and dream things up. You're the one with the unique perspective that leads to new ideas.

Then again, you may never make money at all. That's OK. Do I need to preach to you about the ills of materialism? Haven't you ever regretted the urge to buy, buy, buy? Do you like being a slave to the Great American Commercial? Here is your chance for the eloquently simple life. It's been handed to you on a platter. There is an entire movement called 'Voluntary Simplicity.'

Eddie puts his escape from materialism this way:

> "Well, it's like this. One thing [special chemistry] has done, is it has definitely cured me – 'cured' would be extreme. I would say it has 'astonishingly diminished' my control-

freak-ism. So most people that I see, in our culture, especially this city, are complete and utter control freaks.

> "...And they absolutely believe they have a right to [extreme luxuries], and that's normal. And the control-freak-ism manifests itself in kind of painting really vast luxury – by world standards – by painting it as minor necessities, that one could barely ask for less. [Laughter] There was an ad on Craig's List just two days ago that I read...the woman said, 'Can't I find a normal guy who can take a few months off to travel to [Egypt, Stockholm, anywhere]...? I mean, is that a big deal now, or what? What does a girl have to do to just find a stand-up guy? My God!' So that was the tone of her ad."

Eddie himself has an extremely elegant life, despite strict poverty. He buys only the things he really wants the most, and he searches as long as he has to for good quality at the best price. His apartments always have an air of carefully chosen and arranged articles that are all loved and appreciated. By contrast, my house full of stuff looks unconsidered and indiscriminate.

The point is that now your goals will proceed from your personality, not from someone's idea about what you should be doing. What's wrong with that? Sally sees this as a natural process of growth.

> "People go, 'Oh, how am I going to find the love of my life?' Well, go to the place where you feel most yourself. [Where] you feel most in touch with who you are, that part of you that you really love, that's where you'll find that."

There's a quote from Shirley MacLaine's <u>Dance While</u> <u>You Can</u> that sums it all up for me. "When you're a person to whom money means little, to whom power is burdening, and to whom fame is an invasion of privacy, *success has to be defined by different criteria*" (italics mine).

Then again, you may choose to look on your joblessness as a well-earned retirement. Maybe you don't want a second career. That is OK too. Perhaps the important thing to you in life is having great friendships. You now have time to cultivate them in full. Or simply enjoy life in any one of the hundreds of ways people do. You can walk, you can see, you can attend the myriad events that life provides, you can explore the countryside for miles around by bus and on foot, and be a free spirit. In other words: have a full life! There is nothing on earth that says you have to spend your days with a bag of chips in front of the TV just because you no longer work nine to five.

Jessica describes the little things that bring quality to her life:

> "You need to be doing something, you know…going to school helps. I know that volunteering has helped…Sometimes quality can be just taking a nap when you need it. Sometimes it's really small stuff that just keeps you from losing it…when I get this busy it's hard for me to take my nap because I don't have enough time. And then I start feeling really – you know. 'Now what?' you know? 'There we go, another day, I feel like crap – lovely'. Naps are really important. Just rest is really important.

> "And then there's other things too, quality-wise…I like stuff like just taking walks. Or going to a bookstore and look at all the books and maybe choose one and maybe not. Maybe just deciding which one I'd choose if I *did* feel like buying a book. Stuff like that. Going into shops, walking around. I walk in

urban scenes more than nature. I tend to feel
more comfortable in urban settings. Stuff like
that. Just little things sometimes."

Maybe at one time you wanted power over others. But as
a PASC individual, you can't afford that. What kind of power
can you wield while psychotic? The power of a general over his
soldiers' lives? The power of a surgeon at the operating table?
The power of a CEO over millions of dollars of merchandise
and hundreds of people?

The power of the PASC is that you will finally,
irrevocably, become an individual, following your own unique
path. True individuals do not hunger for power over others
(though they may end up as leaders). They may end up with
money, but they will probably find it outside the nine-to-five
system, in their own particular way. You are no longer one of
the crowd, though there are plenty of others like you. You are
no longer a cog in the system, though the system has made
some provision for you.

What I am trying to say is that you have been given not
just a burden but also a gift.

Maybe that sounds crazy (and we've already established
that I am). But I am not the only one who feels this way.

Sally says:

> "I think I am a sensitive channel, now
> that I'm into that. So I realize it's all
> perspective when it comes to a mystery. I
> choose the perspective that makes me peaceful
> and happy. I'm glad I have choice.

> "It's all about perspective...I believe I
> have a great destiny lined up. I believe I will
> have important work.

> "This society pathologizes it, but I see
> what I have as a gift."

Let me tell you a real-life story.

There was a poor white cracker's son named Ernest Tubb. He wanted to be a singer. Specifically, he wanted to sing in the famous yodeling style of the admired hillbilly singer Jimmy Rodgers. So he sang, and meanwhile dug ditches and drove beer delivery trucks for a living. He had a 15-minute radio show that wasn't going much of anywhere. The yodeling style of hillbilly songs was very difficult to do, but Jimmy had done it first, and better.

Rodgers died in 1933, and in 1936 Tubb moved close enough to visit Rodger's widow and offer his respects. She got him a recording contract with RCA, but still nothing happened. Then in 1939 he had a tonsillectomy.

Now, a tonsillectomy is usually a minor operation. You just do what the doctor tells you, and you'll be fine. But Ernest didn't do that. He sang while recovering, and singing is almost as hard on the voice as yelling. As a result his voice was ruined. He couldn't yodel anymore.

This is where the story gets interesting. He did NOT stop singing, but turned to writing songs for the singing style that was left to him. The new voice was "rougher, yet allowed him to project depth, honesty, and heart *and rescued him from the dead end of being a mere Rodgers clone*" (Italics added. Ernest Tubb, The Definitive Collection by Rich Kienzle).

It was only after this that his career took off. He became a star. He was in the first Grand Ole Opry show ever to play Carnegie Hall. He sang the version of "Blue Christmas" that inspired Elvis Presley. In 1950 he had a hit that crossed over into the Pop Top Ten. And he was allegedly instrumental in getting the name of his music category changed from 'hillbilly' to 'country and western.'

You may never have heard of Ernest Tubb. But you've probably heard of some of the people he gave a leg-up to: Hank Williams, Patsy Cline, Johnny Cash, and Loretta Lynn, just to name a few. The music world would have been different if Tubb had not suffered from the 'disaster' of losing his voice.

I think we can do something like that.

Would I like to be cured? Sure, I would. It would remove a lot of obstacles. But if I could live my life over again, would I live it without ever having special chemistry? *No, I would not!*

Being PASC has given me far too much, taught me too many precious things, for me to ever regret it.

Even Shanna, at 14 years old, knows she has received something special from her struggles.

> "When you pretty much have to fight
> for your sanity, you mature. Nobody's forced
> me to go through the things I went through,
> really. But I went through them myself."

No one can tell you how to proceed from here. You have been forced to create your own story. You can create it any way you want *except* in the common way. You have just made a huge spiritual and evolutionary jump forward, if you care to take advantage of it.

Don't waste it. Be yourself, in the hours you get to choose. That's the road to your best health and contentment.

APPENDIX ONE

Selected Resources:

Just for Fun: *I recommend a series of five novels by Abigail Padgett. The heroine, Bo Bradley, is Bipolar, and gains some of her best hunches and personal qualities from that part of her personality. It helps her solve hair-raising situations in her job as a child services worker.*

The books are: Child of Silence, Strawgirl, Turtle Baby, Moonbird Boy, and The Dollmaker's Daughters.

I would like to think that novels featuring the PASC as protagonists will become more frequent in the book lists. Maybe I'll even write one myself.

A New Concept:

International Center for Clubhouse Development

The Clubhouse movement started in New York in 1994. Now there are 400+ centers around the globe. Each Clubhouse is a center where members can go to socialize during weekends and evenings, participate in decision-making and running of the center, and learn skills that ready them for a Transitional Employment Program during the week. The work is voluntary, members choose their own jobs and work hours, and membership is free. Clubhouses also help support members who want to get further education, and help them access community resources and affordable housing. The statistics of their success are impressive.

After touring my local center, I have decided to join. I wish to work in their multi-media lab and help catalog their new library of donated books.

You can look them up at www.iccd.org
To find out if there is a center near you, visit www.iccd.org/search_form.php

Or write to:

International Center for Clubhouse Development
425 West 47th Street
New York, NY 10036
Phone: 212-582-0343
Fax: 212-397-1649

National Organizations (in alphabetical order):

American Psychiatric Association
1000 Wilson Blvd, Suite 1825
Arlington, VA 22209

703-907-7300
www.psych.org

American Psychological Association
750 First Street NE
Washington, DC   20002

Americans with Disabilities Act
Disability Rights Section Mailing
US Department of Justice
950 Pennsylvania Avenue NW
Civil Rights Division
Disability Rights Section – NYA
Washington, DC 20530

800-514-0301 (voice)
800-514-0383 (TDD)
www.ada.gov

Anxiety Disorders Association of America
8730 Georgia Avenue, Suite 600
Silver Spring, MD 20910

240-485-1001
www.adaa.org

**Center for the Study of Issues
in Public Mental Health**
Nathan S. Kline Institute for Psychiatry
140 Old Orangeburg Road
Orangeburg, NY 10962

845-398-5500
http://csipmh.rfmh.org

Depression and Bipolar Support Alliance
(formerly National Depressive and Manic Depressive Association)
730 North Franklin, Suite 501
Chicago, IL 60610

800-826-3632
312-642-0049
www.ndmda.org OR (newer)
www.dbsalliance.org

Depression and Related Affective Disorders Association
8201 Greensboro Drive, Suite 300
McLean, VA 22102

703-610-9026
888-288-1104
www.drada.org

Depression FAQ (frequently asked questions)
www.mcmanweb.com/depressionfaq.htm

Erase the Stigma
c/o Mental Health America
4069 – 30th Street
San Diego, CA 92104

619-543-0412

Health Care Financing Administration
Dept. of Health & Human Services
200 Independence Avenue SW
Washington, DC 20201

410-786-3000
www.hhs.gov

Internet Depression Resource List
www.marthalakecov.org/~charlatn/depression/resources.html

Internet Mental Health
www.mentalhealth.com

Job Accommodation Network
P.O. Box 6080
Morgantown, WV 26506

800-526-7234 (voice)
877-781-8403 (TTY)
www.bu.edu/cpr

Mental Health America
2000 N. Beauregard St., 6th Floor
Alexandria, VA 22311

703-684-7722
www.nmha.org

National Alliance for Research on Schizophrenia & Depression
60 Cutter Mill Road, Suite 404
Great Neck, NY 11021

800-829-8289
www.narsad.org

National Alliance for the Mentally Ill
(NAMI)
2107 Wilson Blvd., Suite 300
Arlington, VA 22201

703-524-7600
800-950-NAMI
www.nami.org

NAMI works on legislation for the PASC, among other things.
They also have a new website, www.strengthofus.org, for teens,
which is a social network and space for young PASC to talk, blog,

and have fun in all the ways that one can electronically.

National Anxiety Foundation
3135 Custer Drive
Lexington, KY 40517
www.lexington-on-line.com

National Council for Common Behavioral Healthcare
12300 Twinbrook Parkway, Suite 320
Rockville, MD 20852

301-984-6200
www.thenationalcouncil.org

National Institute of Mental Health (NIMH)
Information & Inquiries Branch
6001 Executive Blvd
Bethesda, MD 20892

301-443-4513
1-866-615-6464
www.nimh.nh.gov

Please note that for virtually every diagnosis there is a separate department at NIMH. You can get free pamphlets and up-to-date information here on your diagnosis.

National Mental Health Consumer's Self-Help
1211 Chestnut Street, Suite 1207
Philadelphia, PA 19107

215-751-1810
800-553-4539
www.mhselfhelp.org

National Mental Health Info Center
P.O. Box 42557
Washington, DC 20015

1-800-789-2647
866-889-2647 (TDD)
www.mentalhealth.org

National Organization for Seasonal Affective Disorder
www.nosad.org

National Stigma Clearinghouse
245 – 8th Avenue, # 213
New York, NY 10011

212-255-4411
www.stigmanet.org

Obsessive-Compulsive Foundation
P.O. Box 961029
Boston, MA 02196

617-973-5801
www.ocfoundation.org/what-is-ocd.html

Obsessive-Compulsive Information Center
Madison Institute of Medicine
7617 Mineral Point Road, Ste 300
Madison, WI 53717

608-827-2470
www.miminc.org/aboutocic.html

Obsessive-Compulsives Anonymous
P.O. Box 215
New Hyde Park, NY   11040

516-739-0662
obsessivecompulsivesanonymous.org

Psych Central – Mental Health Infosource
Psych Central
55 Pleasant St, Suite 207
Newburyport, MA   01950

978-992-0008
www.psychcentral.com

Schizophrenia – Doctor's Guide to the Internet
www.docguide.com/news/content.nsf/patientresallcateg/schizophrenia

These are just a few of the many national organizations available to us. You will also find smaller, more regional organizations with just a little digging.

APPENDIX TWO

Special Report

Whose God?

Dealing with Philosophical, Theological, and Scientific Issues in Twelve-Step Programs
by Mel C. Thompson

Part One

1. Introduction

I come to this project with rather specific credentials. In addition to having received a B.A. in Philosophy from a very demanding Department at Cal-State Fullerton in 1982, I am also a person in recovery, have worked Twelve-Step programs, and have suffered from chronic psychiatric problems all of my life.

One problem that often comes up for those looking at a Twelve-Step program, especially with psychiatric problems, is how to confront Steps 2, 3, and 11, though more specifically Step 3, which in a way encompasses the other two.

With globalization, mass media and multiculturalism, working a Twelve-Step program can be confusing once the issue arises of "Turning our wills and our lives over" – or some phrase like it – "...to a Higher Power, as we understood that Higher Power." However we fiddle with the exact wording or nomenclature, we are still presented with this one central problem: how are we to deal with the thorny issues of theology and philosophy that raise their heads?

For the person just starting a recovery program, or even for seasoned Twelve-Steppers trying to carry the message to others, these issues can become a stumbling block. One of the main reasons for this is a lack of education in basic Metaphysics from the philosophical side, and a lack of basic understanding of World Religions from the theological side. There is no exact solution that will work for everyone, whether "joining" the program or "spreading the word" about the program. But I remain optimistic that people can be taught the basics of the metaphysics of others in such a way as to make the program adaptable to each faith (or perceived lack of it). My purpose here will be to provide a crash course in such a way that the program can work from many points of view. This was the intention of the Founders and should remain our intention today.

There is something profoundly more complex with a dual-diagnosis situation (profound psychiatric illness combined with an overt addiction), and philosophical problems for this combined condition can become more perplexing. For reasons I do not fully understand, it seems that psychiatric patients have a special connection with theology and philosophy, and so for them the usually tricky issues of how to accept or connect with "God as we understood God" are even more confusing. We included this section in this book because we found the issue simply needed deeper treatment, particularly for dual-diagnosis patients.

2. What did the Founder believe?

Before I get too deep into the specific problems of philosophy and theology and the conflicts people have about going into a Twelve-Step program, we need to confront the rumors about the religious status of the main Twelve-Step Founder, Bill W.

I have seen in writing and heard people speaking in person and on the radio about Bill W. And the rumor, whether true or false, is often put out that Bill W. was a born-again Christian and that the Twelve-Step program is really a kind of evangelical Christianity in disguise. To make matters more confusing, there is indeed some conceptual overlap between the two, and while the Twelve-Step program does give almost unlimited latitude regarding what a practitioner may or may not believe, the problem for others is that Bill W. often spoke like a Christian, is rumored to have attended Christian churches, and that his program when viewed from a certain light might seem to be leaning in that direction.

One of the cornerstones of evangelical born-again Christianity is a certain Orthodoxy that does not permit diversity of belief. Put simply, Christian Fundamentalism states that there is only one way to be saved from the fires of Hell. So on the face of it, it cannot be possible for the Twelve-Step program to be Orthodox, because the program's main tenet is that *no ONE understanding of God may be used to represent the program as a whole.*

While a born-again Christian is very welcome to become an active Twelve-Step member, s/he is specifically not welcome to use the recovery programs to spread his or her understanding of God. So if Bill W. was a Fundamentalist, he was an odd one, since he founded a worldwide program in which one is blatantly forbidden to dominate the Twelve-Step culture.

3. For the curious: more about Bill W.

For some folks the preceding reassurances are not enough to make them comfortable. Some say there is simply too much Christian language, even if it is "defanged" or watered down. I've not found mention of Bill W. attending any Catholic churches, nor Jewish synagogues, nor Islamic mosques, nor the temples of any Asian religion. The organized religion he had been known to take part in was a very liberal Protestantism. There is little doubt that he attended moderate-to-liberal Protestant churches in his life, but these churches tended to be influenced by the so-called "Pietism" of the time, a movement that stressed ethical purity rather than dogmatic theology.

Even in some so-called Evangelical churches there is a liberal wing called the Dispensationalists. These are Orthodox Christians who are generally conservative and dogmatic in their theological approach. And they may even be given to telling folks that there is only one way to be saved; however, on further cross-examination they will admit that God may have made exceptions and that through some mystery we cannot understand, even a non-Christian or two might be saved through some other religion.

Whether or not Bill W. was a true liberal Protestant or a more Conservative Dispensationalist, one thing is clear. His theology clearly admitted salvation, enlightenment, nirvana, and/or deliverance from addiction and codependency for people of faiths that were specifically not Christian. Without some form of Liberalism or Dispensationalism, it would have been intellectually impossible for Bill W. to found the steps and traditions as he did. In short, a Christian who invites me to his church but says that he encourages me to stick with Hinduism or Islam if it makes me comfortable, or who actually says that my disbelief in God is also welcome and that my Agnosticism will be warmly greeted – well, this person simply cannot be a garden-variety Fundamentalist. And so, while such speculation is considered dangerous, and while this topic is shyly avoided in most Twelve-Step contexts, it should be finally said without qualification that Bill W. was not cut of the same cloth as what we now call Evangelical Born-Again Christianity. It isn't logically possible; and it isn't theologically or philosophically realistic to suppose that he was.

4. What we will do here

While the preceding paragraphs may seem reassuring to some of our religion-phobic brethren, it brings up another problem for those who are not made queasy and are not angered or otherwise brought to some digestive disorder regarding the topic of religion. And this problem, simply put, is: what is an ordinary person with no religion and no philosophical training to do when asked to "turn your will and your life over to a Higher Power"? So while there are some folks who don't want to hear anything about religion, there are some who want to be *given* a religion. And, uncomfortably for these types, the Twelve Steps will neither ban religion nor hand you a specific deity to believe in. Since Agnostics and Atheists who wish to remain so are welcome into the program, and since Muslims, Christians, and Jews of fervent belief are also welcome, how is a newcomer with uncertain convictions and no current affiliation to know what to do?

The difficulty is that the unaffiliated, currently in the throes of addiction, mental illness, or both, and seeking help from a Higher Power, must move forward while not yet necessarily knowing where they will end up. The number of possibilities between these poles is nearly unlimited, and the soul seeking help is then having to make up his or her mind about what to believe the Universe is even made of – one God, several gods, no gods, a Cosmic Force, Karma, life after death, no life after death, and a whole mass of sticky, uncomfortable, often unanswerable questions.

The good news is that there are very sane, very well-known and pleasantly reassuring ways for the Agnostic, the Atheist, the Hindu, the Christian, the Scientist, the Pagan, and the Shaman all to work this great Twelve-Step program.

Also it must be understood – and the program will help you understand this as never before – that the World is often working through us in ways we can't predict; or as an Atheist might say, Evolution is working through each animal. This is the law of unintended consequences. A person attempting to invade a country may find that the country he invaded has culturally taken over his own country.

So Bill W. could have started AA for any reason he liked, but he had no way to control what it would become. And one thing is for sure: A.A. and its affiliated programs are not a vehicle for Christian doctrine. In fact, to the dismay of many organized religions, A.A. has empowered certain people to become theologically and philosophically independent. Many in A.A. and other Twelve-Step programs are, for the first time in their lives, really thinking independently; coming to their own understanding of God and/or the Universe.

In the following pages I will attempt to familiarize the reader with little or no training as to what a World View can be. We will discuss the basic categories that form the world views of almost everyone on the planet, whether consciously or unconsciously. Within this very short outline, you will see World View systems that include religious, non-religious, and even anti-religious viewpoints which may correlate closely to your own. I will suggest possible modes of interaction with the Twelve Steps in such a way that the hesitant reader might see how he or she might find a home within the Twelve Steps and traditions.

Who knows? What you do with the program may lead to developments that no one has foreseen. The program is yours. You decide how you participate, the level of your participation, and you – and only you – decide what your participation means.

Part Two

1. Defining Sanity and Recovery – and 'God'

A very important point to keep in mind as we approach Steps 1, 2 and 3 is that the phrase 'restored to sanity' could actually be a problem for a lot of folks with varying philosophical and diverse religious backgrounds.

Firstly, as our author has mentioned, full restoration to sanity is not even remotely possible for many of us. So the restoration may be looked at as dealing with a secondary effect, being sane about being insane.

As for my own Step 3, which involves learning to trust one's Higher Power as one understands It/Him/Her/Them, a great life-changing realization came over me in reference to 'restoration to sanity.' I discovered that since insanity was my regular state, what needed to be restored to me was a sane way of dealing with my insanity. I am very serious on this point, not only because of its profound effect on recovery itself, but because of some important multicultural and religious diversity issues I plan to discuss.

It may come as a surprise to some of our readers to know that what the typical western scientific outlook calls 'insane' is not insane for many cultures and specifically not for many religions. So we have to be careful when we offer folks a 'restoration to sanity' within our program. In fact, to turn our focus back to Step 1, I'd rather say that I like the term 'manageability' ("We saw that our lives had become unmanageable"). Often Twelve-Step practitioners and literature make the culturally insensitive mistake in assuming that their kind of sanity is the sort of sanity that all people should be restored to.

But as Western ideas move East and Eastern ideas move West, we have to realize that a lot of people facing dual-diagnosis will be doing so as believers in Shamanism. Or they may be witch doctors, warlocks, witches, temple prostitutes, and sacred sexual healers, perhaps even Satanists. In California, as I write this, not only are such faiths gaining ground, they are becoming big-time enterprises involving major press and media. Add to this the fact that UFO religion or some of its central doctrines are embraced, to some degree, by tens of millions of Americans, and one realizes that for us to 'carry the message to those who still suffer,' we're going to have to allow for different kinds of sanity. We're going to have to face the fact that some folks will never be what a western scientific doctor would call sane, but we can hope that they will come to a place where they can manage their relationship with this rather narrowly focused society.

California especially has vast groups of immigrants from parts of Asia, and parts of the Southwest have considerable contingents of believers in Native American indigenous faiths. We could even be faced with considering the position of a person who might be from the Caribbean, perhaps a Rastafarian who may hold what we might think of as a marijuana addiction to be a sacred pursuit.

It is easy for those of us who have been in recovery a long time to feel that we have a solid picture of the recovering addict or mentally ill person. This is where it's important to focus on goals. This is also why 'hitting bottom' (in our addiction or illness) is so important. Hitting bottom brings the sufferer to a place where they define for themselves how they would like their lives to work – and how they don't want it to look any more. Within these bounds we can more easily find our own Higher Power. We allow the sufferers among us to define how sanity would look for them, and how their Higher Power as they understand It/Him/Her/Them could bring them to a place of manageability (a term I'm much preferring to 'sanity').

Additionally, if a person has a very hard-core belief system, we have to respect that. For instance, a Shaman who "receives direction from a cosmic lizard" every day in order to do his work could not attain a state we call sanity even if attempting to recover from cocaine and/or on psychiatric medicines. But we can open our minds far enough to say, "Well, while you're being a Shaman, all this is fine: but you can't act that way at your insurance job." So while our characterization of 'sanity' may not be an option, sanity at work as their boss narrowly defines it may be available. This is where we must trust the sufferers to define what their recovery goals are. One thing is for sure. They cannot feel welcome to turn their will and their lives over to a Higher Power if we say their Higher Power is odd or evil or frightening. Hindus, for instance, can change their presiding deities. Who says there's only one?

Additionally, there are groups of Hindus who still practice smoking as a major religious tenet. In many parts of India one can see very holy priests smoking bowls of hash and other similar substances. Some Native American sects still practice the art of peyote consumption. So for them hallucinations are not tragic, but rather, possibly, a goal.

Even psychiatric science has yet to grasp the import of this: how critical the self-definition of Higher Power, and how important the self-definition of sanity is going to be. Already large hospitals on the East Coast have had to open up Alternative Medicine wings, as has, by the way, our Federal Government (the funding for this part of the NIH was not merely the idea of 'a liberal lunatic' but was and is heavily cosponsored by powerful Republicans, surprisingly). From right to left, there is going to be less agreement about what sanity, sobriety, and recovery are. Diverse ideas exist also on the conservative side. One need only realize that most Pentecostal and Snake-Handler forms of Christianity are populated largely by conservative voters.

Bill W. no doubt saw some of this coming. He was far ahead of his time. We must take the intent of his original vision and think about including everyone humanly possible.

When discussing Twelve-Step programs with others, we need to be aware that we don't really know what most people believe. Even if we have formal education in the religion or philosophy in question, no one is aware of all the splinter groups that exist. There are some forms of Islam that resemble Zen Buddhism. There are forms of Buddhism that resemble fundamentalist Christianity. There are forms of Atheistic Communism that resemble religion.

The key here is to always be ready not to know. Many mystics have talked of not-knowing as a semi-divine state. The idea here is to be very alert, and not jump to any conclusions, even if they've said things that make us sure. It is important to restate, as I will several times, that there are forms of Atheism that are quite religious in their texture and feel, and forms of religion that are quite irreligious in their final effects.

Not only might we not know what a person's faith really is, but they may not know either. I have met plenty of conservatives who in their daily lives are more liberal than most liberals ever dream. And I've known many self-declared liberals whose daily affairs seem to be the most staunchly conservative. As we seek to 'bring the message to those who still suffer,' let's keep in mind that we can't be sure what the program of others will look like. Indeed, some people may start their own groups within a framework of ideas that we never imagined.

Having made these points, I want to get a bit more specific about the various major world views, and how they might see their own Higher Power(s). This is important for those who might one day be program sponsors of people with different notions of how the cosmos functions.

2. Buddhism

So what, for example, would a Zen Buddhist Higher Power look like? It's an interesting question, since most of the Zen Buddhist temples I've gone to don't seem to have any particular type of prayer; nor do they necessarily believe in a presiding Deity. And yet I have known my share of Zen Buddhist alcoholics. So now what?

Some Zen Buddhists, when they are willing to put any label on their faith (and often they aren't), might say that the goal of all beings is to find their Buddha Nature. The idea is that all things in existence don't so much have a God that rules over them, but they do have a Fundamental Nature or Original Nature that remains undiscovered or unfulfilled.

The Founders would have surely meant for the Twelve Steps to include Zen Buddhists. So then I think, to use Constitutional language, the "Framers" would have intended for the Zen Buddhist to use his or her own language when dealing with each of the steps.

In the Steps on our personal inventory the original words say, "Humbly asked God to remove our personal character defects." But we could just as easily say, "Humbly turned to our Buddha Nature within for relief from egotistical deeds and thoughts."

In some schools of Buddhism there are even more direct forms of prayer. One can, for instance, in sects that teach the existence of Bodhisattvas, turn to that Buddhist Savior Being and request that one's ethical life and one's moral fiber be improved. The Bodhisattvas are said to be Buddhist adepts who keep returning to the world of humankind in order to enlighten beings who still suffer. Thus, the step could also be worded, "Humbly called upon the grace of Bodhisattva Quan Yin for aid in removing my sinful behaviors."

In still other schools of Buddhism, such as Tibetan Buddhism, the Guru is worshipped as a Living Buddha. Such Gurus are said to sense the prayers and callings of their students, even over great times and distances. Perhaps we could say, "Humbly sought the guidance of our Lama for illumination on how to rid myself of these character defects."

In Pure Land Buddhism, the Amida Buddha is said to have attained enlightenment for all personkind such that simply calling out His name turns one's sins into rays of pure light. It would not take much imagination to see how the step in question could be phrased to make it well adapted to that school of Buddhism.

The task of adapting the Twelve Steps could be a bit rougher in terms of Theravada Buddhism with its strong emphasis on total self-reliance. But even so, there is a fellowship in these groups, and there are Priests, and there is a teaching that there is an Original Nature. In such cases it is usually necessary to identify the Higher Power as being a part of one's own Highest Self. People are complex, and it could be that the power to change is within us, but it may not be within our rational or conscious minds. It may even rest with a part of us to which we feel we have no access. And so, in a way, prayer as such may turn out to be simply a way of talking to a part of ourselves that is too big to fit into the rational structure. (This letting go of control, and this trusting of something larger than one's own conscious thoughts, may be what prayer is anyway.) Hence the Zen Buddhist or Theravada Buddhist in meditation, or while chanting, may be accessing – though not through prayer as we think of it – that side of the self that has the power to cure.

The Higher Power need not be celestial or otherworldly or nonmaterial, but it does generally need to be something beyond the usual field of play, beyond the usual thoughts that we have. The Higher Power could possibly be the part of us that does not think but simply IS. It's fair enough to think we can look at our unmanageable lives and seek to bring them to the place within us that is stronger, larger and purer.

3. <u>Hinduism</u>

The majority of people with unidentified belief systems, theologies, and philosophies, without knowing it, subscribe to the general world view of Pantheistic Hinduism. A lot of people proceed through life with this set of underlying assumptions, but never identify them as such. A struggle often happens with these folks as they approach a Twelve-Step program because they don't know how to use their own feeling about the Universe in their recovery.

Many people see the Universe as a singular system emerging out of God, but this brings them a problem with the theistic wording of the step literature. However, this is only because they are unaware of a world view that accommodates both the "personal relationship" aspect of spirituality and the Pantheistic view: that the Universe is not a place ruled over by a god but is rather a vast sacred organism.

According to most Hindus, the cosmos itself is sacred and is not separate from God, but literally is God's body. Pantheism, the view that the Universe is itself God, is certainly quite popular outside of Hindu circles. However, more Western European forms of Pantheism and homegrown American Pantheism tend to be impersonal. If one is worshipping the whole Universe, then there is no particular Person that one can turn one's will and life over to. And so the Western Pantheist can run into trouble because it is hard to imagine how one could surrender one's will to the sky itself or to the ocean, since the world is not an entity to which one could literally talk and with which one could have a relationship.

Theism, the metaphysical system that we are more overtly familiar with in the West, teaches that before the Universe was created, nothing existed except God, who presumably was infinitely alone, and out of nothing, God created a world separate from Himself. Pantheism proposes that the whole Universe always existed; always was one vast sacred organism or Unity; and that all that we see and don't see and all that was and is and will be are the Body of God. In Theism, the world, the cosmos
, the universe (all without capital letters) are in fact not God and are eternally separate from His being. Often with people who are rather vague in their own beliefs, there is an underlying conflict that no one can quite identify. This conflict is usually between a rather subconscious Theism or a subconscious Pantheism.

In any case, the Hindus arrived at a beautiful solution for all of this. They simply declared that it's *all true*. The entire Universe is the Body of God; however, the entire universe could also be one vast Person inside of whose body we live and with whom we form the Unity that is the whole Universe. Within this wide context God (the Universe) can also appear as a personal God, or millions of personal gods. And God can also appear as a woman, or an animal, or a mountain. So Hindu Polytheism is literally one with Hindu Pantheism. All of the Gods are really one God, and all of the Universe, including ourselves, are literally the body of that God.

In Hinduism, one is free to choose a form or manifestation of God with whom one forms a relationship. It's understood that this exact form of God is not the only possible form of God, since God is literally everything that He, She, or It can appear as. The believer may approach the Infinite Unity from whatever angle works for them.

This really might be true to the spirit of "God as we understood God." In Hinduism, if you understand God to be a woman, you worship Kali or Parvati or Laxmi or Sita. If you understand God to be an animal, you worship Hanuman or Ganapati. If you understand God to be a man, you worship Indra or Krishna. And if God seems androgynous to you, Shiva may seem appealing. There is no time to go into the almost infinite permutations of Hinduism here. A Hindu Twelve-Step practitioner can approach the Universe through an almost countless number of manifestations, picking one or two – or a dozen – that have the most magnetic force.

Each of the gods of Hinduism really refer to some part of the larger Universe, *but approached from one specific angle.* Brahma is the Creator God, Vishnu is the Sustainer God, and Shiva is the Destroying God and the Seed for the coming creation, and Mother Kali is Time itself. Depending on how one is feeling about life and the Universe, the cosmos, while technically impersonal and non-theistic, can nonetheless be approached personally and Theistically in a qualified sense.

I don't know what, if anything, the Founders of the Twelve-Step programs knew about Hinduism, but I've often suspected that they had a subconscious sense of this approach: that is to say, a God manifest in as many different ways as there are people to perceive God. In this way, one could say Hinduism has six billion gods and the Twelve-Step practitioner, if they have leanings this way, can choose any one of them.

4. <u>Taoism And The Organic World View</u>

As Alan Watts used to say, "Taoism views the Universe as an Organism." This is a little different than Hinduism, because Taoism, while having many small schools which do include myths and icons, tends to be taken by the world at large as a rather reduced-mythology tradition. One can still find Hindus who have a literal belief in the mythology of Hinduism, even if they are in the minority; however, in Taoism, one would be hard pressed to find too many folks hanging onto any of the myths as literal truths. The myths themselves, which are barely included in the main scriptures, don't lend themselves to historical claims. For this reason, Taoism is very much studied the world over, as its concepts don't seem so attached to any particular culture or time.

Taoism teaches that Yin and Yang are really two sides of one force, the Great Flow of the Universe. The Universe is seen as a place of balance, where even excessive goodness must be corrected by a dose of evil. The cosmos   has a duty to keep in balance in all ways. There is not much of a teaching of sin, nor even much emphasis on error in Taoism, but mostly a concern to explain the working of the Universe and how It balances itself out. The hope is that people can stop resisting the laws of the Cosmic activity but learn to surf the waves of change; hence the now ubiquitous saying, "Go with the flow," a concept almost certainly rooted in the importation of Taoist concepts.

It's a bit harder to integrate Taoism into the Twelve Steps. But when we get around to Step Two, we can see a possible application. Since we, "Came to believe that a Power greater than ourselves could restore us to sanity," we may have noticed our previous, or even current, Us-against-the-World sense of things. People with profound emotional and chemical imbalances are often the products of environments and /or biochemistries that almost preclude the hope of getting basic needs met.

One reason I have often been so jealous and bitter against healthy folks is that they usually get off on a good footing and learn the basic rules of life, and not even consciously, but subconsciously. When one starts out in a healthy and well-adjusted system and environment, almost implicit in everything said and done, is a reasonable and tested path. Put another way, there are a lot of Taoists out there who don't know they even practice the principles of Taoism, but they simply seem to know when to play their hand, when to fold their cards, when to come on strong and when to retreat quickly. Similar Chinese philosophy can be found in the I-Ching and the Art of War. And so there are several religions and/or major schools of philosophical thought that deal with how an imbalanced person might stop trying to surf waves that have already broken and stop trying to create waves in a vast, still ocean.

The addicted or mentally ill person is caught up in a vicious cycle of control, manipulation, overcompensation…constantly we see an unnecessary struggle. In one great Taoist scripture (and this refers strongly to Step One) are these words: "Have you heard of the preying mantis who raised its arm to stop an oncoming carriage, not realizing this was beyond its power?" How unimaginably perfect a description of our own struggles in life. Another passage, "Who can wait till the mud settles?" And other passages talk about acting quickly when the right moment comes. The timing of mentally ill people is simply cursed at every moment, because often at the root of the mental illness is the desire to make up for lost time by "finally taking charge," or by "never letting myself be fooled again." Hence, in a mad rush to shove their agenda onto a world that frankly resists all agendas, the mentally ill and the addicted fare horribly and most of their endeavors end up in sheer farcical tragicomic failure.

But when we get to Step Two, the Taoist can have a strong hand, perhaps by coming to believe that the Flow of the Universe (here called a Higher Power) may have more wisdom than we do. And so one great step to recovery can be to change from people who are hounding the Universe for their needs to be met, to people who watch the cosmos and see where the flow is going. So many times I found that my greatest successes, or my greatest deliverances, came at times where I dropped my entire agenda and simply said, "What is happening around me? Is there an opportunity here that I didn't plan on?" And much of the time there is.

To an outsider this may all look very flaky, like someone who, rather than choosing a career, goes with whatever jobs seem most comfortable at the time, or who opts for celibacy instead of dating. Or perhaps several career changes, several changes in housing or other things considered "serious," may be given up or taken on based on kinds of intuitions generally considered taboo. I was, for example, feeling weird and "outside" and alien during one course of therapy, and it was all due to my feeling I had too few friends and almost no lovers and practically no family. I had read so many times that these were all sure signs of very serious downward spirals about which one really should become alarmed. But then my therapist noted, it is not fundamentally a problem to be without much money or to be without many social contacts if it is not a problem for the patient.

The Flow of the Universe may dictate that this should be a quiet and solitary time, and it may be that the happiest course might be to go along with this.

But given our culture, our first reaction is to want to "Envision for ourselves a better life and choose prosperity." Often this ends in us simply   wasting our few remaining dollars on miracle cures or turn-your-life-around-in-a-weekend seminars.

So while the Taoist may be very far from having a personal
God, he may, as Lao Tsu said, "rely on the Great Mother," which is
the "very Flow of the cosmos Itself."

5. <u>Theism Revisited</u>

It practically goes without saying that the Twelve Steps were
originally conceived by a Theist who felt the majority of those
interested in the Twelve Steps would be Theistic, and, as a result, the
original Twelve Steps were written with wording that casually sounds
like a Christian or Muslim or Jew wrote them. Again, the Founder
never intended to exclude those of other world views, and in fact his
intention was to include them. And so it is then good for us to know
what this thing called Theism is, and it is also good for non-Theistic
readers to grasp this so that they can define what they are and are not
doing in the program.

Theism is a world view most commonly associated with
Christianity, Islam, and Judaism, but is by no means restricted to them.
The Bahai Faith is a modern theistic religion, as is Mormonism, the
Jehovah's Witnesses, and also the Ancient Zoroastrians were Theistic.
So what is it that separates Theism from other faiths? What are its
main characteristics, and why does it appear to be so popular and so
dominant in world history?

To state it plainly, Theism teaches that the world was created
by a God absolutely and eternally separate from the world and all
beings in it. According to Theism, the world was not created from a
part of God, but was created literally out of nothing, called into
existence from nowhere. And thus, according to Theism, all of nature
and every animal, and every other spiritual entity is distinctly not God.
God exists in a kind of metaphysical isolation according to this world
view. It is sometimes called dualism, although not so accurately, by
those who want to point out that in Theism the cosmos has two types
of being, non-God stuff, and God, and the two can never be one
substance or one being.

One of the reasons why this view of the world is so popular is
because, although it sounds a bit technical at first, it's actually very
easy when one is trying to keep one's story straight, and especially

when one needs help. Hinduism, and in a different way, Taoism, and to some extent certain Native American faiths, are very cloudy as to who exactly is responsible for what, since, in some sense, they teach that the whole of nature emerged, or is currently a part of, the body of God. This makes the concept of sin a murky one. An obvious question a Theist can ask a Non-Theists is, "How can someone do wrong, since all that is done is actually done by some part of God, simply in another form?"

Theism makes prayer a very simple matter. We are praying to an entity above us who is in control, and to an entity who is definitely outside of us, exterior to us, to whom we can appeal for help in a very personal-sounding way. One problem with Pantheism, when it comes to prayer is this: If all beings are a part of God, and therefore, in some sense, God Himself / Herself, then isn't a prayer a part of God asking another part of God for help? It may seem far-fetched, but this is what the Bhagavad-Gita suggests. And too, do not we already talk to ourselves? Do we not already, when dealing with an illogical part of ourselves, refer the question or issue at hand to a more logical or stronger part of ourselves? Clearly, if a single person could be of such a divided mind, it stands to reason that some parts of the Universe are not as enmeshed in the great drama as other parts are.

So Hinduism provides a way for the person in trouble, who according to some types of Hinduism is really a part of God lost in his own vast Epic drama of creation. The myth goes that God, alone in the Universe, is engaged in what we call "suspension of disbelief," enjoying his own story/drama.

This is the same power that allows us to watch a show and become really lost in it to the point of becoming emotional, although we actually know, in another part of ourselves, that the play is not real. The miracle of suspension of disbelief, and no one can explain this yet, is that humans are capable of simultaneously believing in something to the point of emotional exhaustion, while at the same time 100% knowing it not to be real. If God has this power too, and there is no reason He or She or It could not, then indeed, a character in God's play could pray to the Universe and be heard by the part of God in the play, and indeed this is the way hundreds of millions of people look at prayer, although few Westerners really grasp this.

Theism, however, is a bit more popular than Pantheism because the theory of God engaging in a suspension of disbelief in order to create the universe is avoided. God, according to Theism, is not truly lost in His own play. (Christianity does have some hints of such a possibility, although when this gets discussed too frequently, the topic can find itself off limits.) In any case, Theism is a great faith for people in crisis because they know they are small beings in a big universe ruled by and created by another entity, who will be in charge.

The Pantheist looking at a Twelve Step program has a bit of a trickier time. He or she will have to accept that the part of the Universe each of us plays is the part of a lost person finding his or her way home – which is, after all, the great theme of Pantheism: all the little parts of God finding their way back home to the great God in whose being they all share. It's a cyclic expansion and contraction of the cosmos. The alcoholic Pantheist, the sex-addict Pantheist and the dual-diagnosis Pantheist can recognize that the Prodigal Son or Daughter role has reached an end, and the time to return to the Center of All Being has come.

Again, no such fancy footwork, nor literary adroitness is required for the Theist. God is safely 'not us.' And the universe is also 'not God.' By the way, Polytheism and Pantheism often mix well, since the Polytheist, sometimes seeing the entire Universe as God, will decide that each element in nature is a god, and all gods are a part of the Big God, which is everything. Hence the Polytheist can be seen praying to the ocean, or to the wind, since they are all gods, a part of The One.

For some folks in crisis, this is not acceptable. They cannot wonder whether they should pray to a tree, a river, their husbands or angels or whomever. So it's often best for them if there is one God in heaven and nowhere else, or a God who is everywhere, but not actually, so to speak, really merged with anything.

In any case, Theism is generally the order of the day for so many folks entering recovery, often in fear of their lives, and this is fine. But we have to keep a sharp eye out for folks who are not buying into the Theism thing, and we need to know what Theism is, so that we can identify Non-Theists and see why they are struggling, and hopefully we can help them to understand that there are more options than they may be aware of. We may even be called upon to do some brainstorming to assist a Non-Theist in adapting the steps to their own journey.

6. <u>Atheism and the Twelve Steps</u>

While use of the Twelve Steps of recovery movements is generally thought to be a kind of nondenominational religious activity, it has been noted that it is possible to construct a program similar to the Twelve Steps without invoking any spiritual powers.

However, before I go into this possibility, I want to inform the reader that atheism is not usually what they believe it is. And, in fact, most self-declared Atheists do not actually accept the philosophical ramifications of Atheism. Most self-proclaimed Atheists are at best Agnostics, or are actually religious in ways which they fail to see. And so before showing how the Twelve Steps can be used in an Atheistic context, I want to spell out exactly what real Atheism is and what it implies, since practically no one outside of professional philosophical circles has a grip on this.

Most people when they declare themselves Atheists mean approximately this: "I was raised in an environment where a particular religion was dominant. I don't like that religion any more and I have not yet formally joined another church." Such a declaration actually amounts to something akin to Agnosticism. Agnosticism is the position that one does not know, or cannot know, or that it is not important to know, whether or not certain spiritual concepts are true. An Agnostic can be a person who has dropped out of formal religious practice and who suspects that there may not be a God. An Agnostic can also be a person from a non-religious family who believes that while there may or may not be a God, or spiritual powers, the main purpose of life is to live for things that can be seen, felt, heard, and touched. An Agnostic can also deeply doubt the existence of God and go so far as to say, "I find it hard to imagine that any kind of Deity exists, and I myself am opposed to virtually all organized religions."

While the foregoing seems to many people to constitute Atheism, in fact such doctrinal statements come nowhere near approaching the severe set of tenets that actually comprise Atheism.

Atheism is known under a few different headings in formal Philosophy, one of which is Naturalism: the belief that there is absolutely nothing existing in this universe, nor any other universe, which is in any way magical, paranormal, spiritual, or non-material. Put another way, Naturalism teaches that only the material or matter found in nature exists, and this matter is only ever acted upon by the mechanical and physical laws of the universe, and no other force whatsoever. Hence, according to Naturalism, no entities, no forces, no powers, no energies and nothing at all mystical in any way has ever at any time in the history of the universe existed, even for an instant. Furthermore, Naturalism teaches that even within non-religious language, many forces and entities are constantly referred to that in fact have no material, mechanical, physical or logical basis in the actual workings of the world we live in.

So many an Atheist will come in fresh from having lambasted the belief that other people may have in invisible entities only to then proclaim how mysterious and wonderful love is, not realizing that there is nothing materially existing in the Naturalistic world view called 'love.' There are brains, and those brains experience, according to Naturalism, certain biochemical states caused by the secretion of certain chemicals and the effects of certain electrical impulses. Those chemical and electrical reactions may be called 'love' by us; however there is not, in true Naturalism, a separate mystical non-physical thing called love which kind of hovers non-materially around human bodies.

This is only one example. The reader will soon see many more, just by watching an avowed Atheist speak. Implied through the speech of most 'Atheists' are non-material states of being and duties elevated to religious-sounding levels – although of course in a universe of merely mechanical reactions no such states could really exist in such poetic ways.

Naturalism is also, in scientific, philosophical, and political circles, called Materialism. Here, I don't mean the kind of materialism we ascribe to a person who shops too much or is greedy for many luxuries. Rather, Materialism is a philosophy which, like Naturalism though even more directly, says that nothing exists in the universe but the stuff, the material, of which the universe consists. There are subatomic particles and electromagnetic waves and varying frequencies of light out of which our physical world is composed. Beyond that, nothing can be real.

So for instance, one could not properly be an Atheist but also believe in Astrology, fortune telling, psychic powers, nor most of Asian or alternative medicine. One could not be a true Atheist and believe in the doctrines that most Yoga teachers espouse. Most forms of meditation would also be highly illogical in an Atheistic context. In fine, a real Atheist, who really is prepared to carry through with the full implications of Atheism, is a rare breed of cat indeed; so rare, actually, that I myself have met very few of them, and I have searched extensively. They do exist, but what we mostly encounter are Agnostics who like the sound of the word 'Atheism' without having any idea how far-reaching the implications of Atheism are.

Now that we have that bit of business out of the way, I go on to the hard task of looking into what Atheists might do if they sought to have a Twelve-Step type of recovery program in their lives. Clearly they would have to rework or reword the Twelve Steps in some way that did not violate their principles.

The first problem is the Higher Power. In Western culture, that Power is generally thought of as an ordinary kind of Theistic Father God figure. Such a concept won't do for an Atheist. However, Atheists I have met deal with the issue this way. They have in one way or the other made 'The program' or 'The Group' their Higher Power. So like the believer in God, the Atheist acknowledges that his or her life has been ruined by an addiction and also admits that life has become unmanageable. They also admit they cannot conquer their addiction alone. The Atheist then turns to the group for support, guidance, and nurturing, the sort that supplies a kind of power that sheer personal will cannot match.

Let us take for instance Step 5, which discusses admitting the exact nature of our wrongs to another human being and to God. While it's true the Atheist has no God to confess these wrongs to, he or she might have an AA sponsor who would be willing to share this burden. From a therapeutic standpoint, persons with or without faith are made stronger when they have someone to tell their story to. An Atheist in recovery who was tempted to drink alcohol would be in a lot safer position if he or she had a member of a recovery group to call. And in this sense, Step 5, even without the element of God, still has great value.

Step 1, the 'admission of powerlessness', is surely a step that can be taken without bringing God into the process.

Steps 2 and 3 are difficult but not impossible to work with. Again the Atheist in recovery could come to believe that working with the recovery group and following the guidelines of the sober lifestyle could restore him or her to sanity. The Higher Power could be viewed as the Program itself, or the group of people working on recovery.

Steps 4 through 10 involve basic personal accountability and responsibility and a willingness to turn one's life around with the help of the Group rather than of God.

Step 11 can be viewed as a vow to keep in contact with whatever or whoever inspired the person to keep away from their former behaviors. Such activities could include working out, going to therapy, working through family problems, visiting peaceful places, and so on.

Step 12 can simply be the urging of all recovering persons to continue to reach out to those who still need help.

So the point of view of Atheism is problematic but not insurmountable. More than anything, a bit of creativity would be required.

7. <u>The Genius of the Twelve Steps</u>

When Bill W. had his own revelation, a revelation that many complain he never fully explained or fully revealed, he did so within our American culture at a time in our culture where, for most of the population, Monotheism was not "a religion," but was "the religion," and it was not "an idea" but simply "obvious truth." Bill W. intuited, however, that the future was soon to be far more complex. And so, some speculate (as I do) that he dealt with the difference between the monocultural reality he faced at the time and the pluralistic culture he knew would soon arrive, by designing the Twelve Steps as – to use a motivationalist term – a "transitional technology."

He also saw that the Twelve Steps, while destined to become famous first in the United States and Europe, was going to be a worldwide phenomenon and that persons who were not Monotheists would eventually need the tools he had to offer. The question remained: how to get this movement going, make the Monotheists all around us comfortable and, at the same time, build in provisions for the non-Monotheistic cultures and ideologies that would soon be all around us?

For the average conservative Christian, Jew, or Muslim, the Twelve Steps seem annoyingly tolerant, but still, they come off with a general Monotheistic tone that creates enough comfort for the theologically orthodox to get on with the program. For persons coming to the Twelve Steps from a conservative Monotheistic background virtually nothing in the Twelve Steps needs to be explained, since, except for the "bothersome tolerance" present in the Twelve Steps, the bulk of it could just as well have been written by a believer in the Bible, the Torah, or the Koran.

The tactical genius of Bill W. is how precisely he threaded the needle in such a way as to gain a vast Monotheistic base from the society around him and, at the same time, create the seed for exporting the program around the world and retaining it, once Monotheism began to be challenged in the United States as it is now by neo-Pagan, Hindu, Taoist, Buddhist, and Humanistic traditions; and also from within, by American-born citizens, as well as by Immigrant citizens coming here from every part of the planet. Their very presence disabuses the average American of the idea that the theological world outside of Monotheism isn't really serious or sizable.

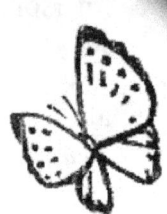